THE THAW

RECLAIMING THE PERSON FOR PSYCHIATRY

Second Edition, Revised and Expanded

PAUL GENOVA, M.D.

With a Foreword by Paul H. Ornstein, M.D.

THE THAW

RECLAIMING THE PERSON FOR PSYCHIATRY

Second Edition, Revised and Expanded

PAUL GENOVA, M.D.

With a Foreword by Paul H. Ornstein, M.D.

Routledge
Taylor & Francis Group
New York   London

First published 2002 by
The Analytic Press, Inc.

This edition published 2013 by Routledge

Routledge   Routledge
Taylor & Francis Group   Taylor & Francis Group
711 Third Avenue   27 Church Road
New York, NY 10017   Hove, East Sussex BN3 2FA

Routledge is an imprint of the Taylor & Francis Group, an informa business

Library of Congress Cataloging-in-Publication Data

Genova, Paul,
    The thaw : reclaiming the person for psychiatry /
Paul Genova ; with a foreword by Paul H. Ornstein.
—2nd ed., rev. & expanded
        p. cm.
    Previously ed. published with subtitle: 24 essays in
psychotherapy.
    Previously ed. published: Pittsburgh, PA : Dorrance,
c2000.
    Includes bibliographical references.
    ISBN 0-88163-380-1
    1. Psychotherapy—Miscellanea.   2. Psychotherapy
—Anecdotes.   3. Psychotherapist and patient—Miscellanea.
I. Title.

RC454.4 .G485 2002
616.89'14—dc21
                                    2002074592

for Library of Congress   98-47700
                                          CIP

Dedication

For the two therapists that I paid...
And two that I didn't: Margaret Nichols and Darrell Dawson.

The goose is frozen in the lake.
I'm going to thaw it out.

The goose was hurt in the wings.
The ice came fast.
The others left without it.
The ice came fast.

I'll build a small fire
by the goose.
Frightened look in its eyes.
See, its neck is stretching
the way the others went.
It's got the south
in its neck,
stretching that way.
But the wings kept it here.
The broken wings.

I'm going to thaw it out.

told by Isaac Greys (Otter Lake, Manitoba)
translated from the Cree by Howard Norman

CONTENTS

FOREWORD

The Thaw is an amazingly refreshing collection of down-to-earth, yet profound writings on a variety of themes, in short-story format, appropriately subtitled "Reclaiming the Person for Psychiatry." These essays are about psychiatry and psychotherapy, to be sure, but they are also about much more. Paul Genova's erudition is impressive; his clinical astuteness even more so. The range of his interests is varied and extensive. His ability to encapsulate in each of his "stories" something essential about clinical realities marks this collection as an extraordinary achievement. The collection is a valuable companion for psychotherapist and general psychiatrist alike—read the stories one at time and let each story percolate in your mind and become a part of you. This collection, now expanded with an additional eight chapters, is well worth a second printing and should reach a larger audience of mental health professionals who did not read these pieces on first publication.

Dr. Genova is a thoughtful, sensitive clinician whose agile mind seems to have extracted from his own clinical experience, from his readings, and from his being attuned to the important issues of the day a sound, practical philosophy for our time. He generously shares with his readers his actual work with patients. Having dared to leave the boundaries of a restricted, theory-centered approach to psychotherapy for a primarily patient-centered approach, he teaches us what I would call the use of a *disciplined spontaneity* in his creatively structured treatment approach. His work is, of course, not without theory—he knows that there is no theory-free observation—but the theory that guides his work is what we often refer to as the private theory of the clinician and not one of the burgeoning formal, public theories of the field. We know that even those who seem to adhere to one of the many formal, public theories, when confronted with the unpredictable individualities of their patients, inevitably resort to their own private, often unarticulated theories; these are the theories that appear to be most responsive to the

ix

idiosyncratic needs of their patients. The stories about the treatment experiences exemplify the therapeutic relationship with concrete examples and thereby articulate these private, otherwise unarticulated theories. This is their greatest merit.

In the tradition I come from, the Hasidic Masters taught with short stories and parables, never explicating them, with the hope that the stories would convey the essence of their teaching without enslaving listeners' minds to the Master's voice. Paul Genova does the same. The short-story format is well suited to his intent to convey to his readers not only what comes from his mind, but, more important, what comes from his clinically sophisticated heart—if that is a permissible phrase.

The stories selected for this volume, many of them originally in journalistic style—here somewhat modified—succeeded in capturing the attention of the readers of *Psychiatric Times* or *Voices*, when they originally appeared. Each successive piece was avidly awaited, because Genova was articulating common concerns that only few of us take the trouble, or have the gift, to put into words and offer to our colleagues. Genova is also an avid reader and has his ears cocked to the ground to be in touch with the rapid changes in our field, and he always responds to such changes as rapidly as journalistic intent demands. The value of Genova's stories and essays, however, resides in their having much more than short-lived journalistic interest. Their content transcends their immediate relevance—they have a message of lasting value, especially in our current antipsychotherapy culture in general and in psychiatry in particular. Nowadays, subjective experience is generally bypassed to the detriment of our patients and ourselves.

Genova's message is a sustained, valiant effort to buck this trend. His courage is to be applauded, his style to be admired. Here, the "provincial rustic" is felicitously fused with the reluctant, sparkling intellectual he wishes to hide—but it shines through in his writings nevertheless.

The title of the book is taken from one of the essays. When I first saw the title, my association was that the content of the volume probably articulates the loosening of the rigidities often prevalent among theory-centered psychotherapists. Before I opened the book, I kept wondering whether its author advocated the currently prevalent approach to psychotherapy, namely, to conduct it without any guiding theory. I found just the opposite. In his definition of what psychotherapy is, he lays down the ground rules for its conduct and foreshadows a disciplined approach. I was also impressed by Genova's approach to treatment; he not only teaches others by example—but, through his writings, he also "teaches" himself by articulating what he has experienced as a therapist. He knows that examples have a more powerful impact than "preaching" about a therapeutic attitude would achieve.

The book is organized in four sections. Genova introduces each section by spelling out the red thread that runs through the individual chapters it contains. Each chapter is again introduced briefly, highlighting the main points and aiding the reader in developing his or her own thoughts as an accompaniment to the author's well-formulated ideas. It is a helpful guide.

The reader may disagree here and there with the approach used in some of the clinical examples or with the attitude exemplified, but that does not detract from this "work in progress." We are all engaged in work in progress throughout our professional lifetime; there is no training that prepares us for the job forever. This book is an aid to reflection as our field and, indeed, the world around us, undergoes rapid change. We value the straightforward description of the clinical process in a literary rendition that allows us to enter into Paul Genova's experiences and empathize with the patient as well as the therapist, to our own enrichment. The job of refining our approach to patients in distress is never finished—it is challenged anew with each therapeutic encounter.

Our profession is enriched not only by Paul Genova's stories and essays, but also by his collegial generosity of spirit. This generosity manifests itself in various ways, none more telling than Genova's giving us all explicit permission to use his ideas to pursue our own—freely but responsibly.

Paul H. Ornstein, M.D.
Professor of Psychoanalyis (Emeritus)
Department of Psychiatry
University of Cincinnati
June 2002

PREFACE

For the past 17 years I have been writing short clinical essays from my psychiatric practice. This activity started as my own means of coping with the rigors of clinical work and with the progressive depersonalization—even de-personing—of the psychiatric profession during this time. In these papers I expressed an anticipatory nostalgia for the kind of practice I was trying to maintain, wherein selves, not brains, remained the fundamental clinical concern, and the uniqueness of every relationship, rather than standardized or orchestrated interactions, remained my most effective clinical tool. Awestruck by the exponential progress of neuroscientific understanding, I nevertheless registered my ambivalence about the simplistic ways in which such knowledge—which has the potential to contribute to an even subtler understanding of persons—devolved into the pharmaceutical algorithms on which my younger colleagues' training was increasingly based.

I found many readers who shared my sentiments as these pieces began to appear in print; my writing continued with their encouragement. I no longer felt alone but, rather, in good company. Some of these papers have been widely read, particularly among psychiatrists, and have even had some small influence on the discourse of the day. Others, including some of my own favorites, were less noticed. In this book I gather some of the best of them together in a more permanent form, thereby giving them a second lease on life—and, I hope, a wider audience among psychotherapists as well as interested general readers.

I am neither a scientist nor a psychological theorist but, rather, a sort of psychiatric journalist; some might say that the word essay overly dignifies these newspaper pieces and journal articles. I use the word in its original sense of "to try": to try to understand myself and my work better by writing about it. My journalist's or essayist's method generates more questions than answers and offers no comprehensive theory or set of techniques. To the extent that I possess either, I would not want to make the slightest suggestion that anyone else should behave or think like me when working with patients. As I often tell trainees, the only reason to learn about someone else's approach, including mine, is to become one's own best kind of therapist.

Being a clinician rather than a theorist, I like my theory rough-and-ready. Grand systems that account for just about everything are too easily mistaken for reality. I mistrust them—I prefer simple and obviously provisional ideas that generate useful questions and so get me started. In this I feel in league with the late American poet Amy Clampitt:

> What I'm really concerned with is maintaining what I have to call a subversive attitude, the opposite of going along with anybody's program whatever. It amounts to wariness about being co-opted. Since part of being co-opted means having to accept somebody else's language, I see this wariness as a particular function of poets.
> —Interview quoted in the
> *London Review of Books*, 2/5/98

That said, it won't be difficult for readers to identify my recurrent intellectual debts to D.W. Winnicott and Carl Jung, James Hillman and Jiddu Krishnamurti, Milton Erickson, and Michael Balint. It has sufficed me to read more deeply than widely; the results of this simple and accessible diet are everywhere apparent.

Psychodynamic psychotherapy of a flexible and tradesmanlike kind has always been at the center of my way of working. Once, while lecturing to a skeptical psychiatric audience about it, I proposed a "poor man's definition" of this time-tested approach. I may as well quote it here in full as a set of orienting premises underlying all the work described in this book.

"Poor Man's Definition of Psychodynamic Psychotherapy"

A narrative and historical approach to human problems that seeks to understand and use an individual story in its own terms and to use a therapeutic relationship in its own *unique* and nonstandardized terms, with the following four assumptions:

1) People want things (drives).
2) People need connection with other people (attachments).
3) People are often *unconscious* of these wants/needs and how their behavior and experience are shaped by them.
4) Developmental history and subsequent life story are important for an understanding of the present, as are genetically based temperament and disease vulnerability.

Most of the essays collected here appeared, in slightly different form, in either *Psychiatric Times*, a widely read professional newspaper, or *Voices*, the official journal of the small but redoubtable American Academy of Psychotherapists (AAP). Those pieces written for *Voices* assume a readership of seasoned therapists and are, as is the journal's custom, quite personal. In the *Psychiatric Times* papers I tried to be an advocate for psychotherapy, and for simple human contact within the wider and fast-changing arena of mainstream American mental health care. Thus, in the *Times* pieces I often entered into the debates of the day and had to reckon with such things as the new, manualized therapy techniques and the nomenclature of the standard *Diagnostic and Statistical Manual of Mental Disorders, 4th Edition* (DSM-IV). I have included such topical essays or passages here only if I judged them to have a wider or more enduring relevance to ongoing issues within the professions of psychiatry and psychotherapy, or indeed to the very idea of psychotherapy itself

I wish you good reading, which is to say that I hope something herein touches, inspires, challenges, provokes, instructs, or at least usefully irritates you.

This book was first published as *The Thaw: 24 Essays in Psychotherapy* by Dorrance Publishing in the year 2000. For this second edition, under the auspices of The Analytic Press, eight more pieces and introductory material for them have been added to the first edition with little or no change in the original structure or approach aside from a new subtitle. My tendency has always been to make the same few simple points in different contexts by coming to them from various directions and often arriving at a place whose familiarity belies the deceptive difficulty of getting there and staying there. I play the same notes, over and over. I hope I have played them better and better.

Lewiston, Maine
March 2002

PART I:
SEVEN VISITATIONS

INTRODUCTION TO PART I

One might imagine that therapy takes place in some timeless intersubjective present, but it doesn't. History and culture lurk just outside the door. Historians teach us, in fact, that the highly individualistic kind of "self" which undertakes, or practices, psychotherapy is a recent and evolving phenomenon and not a universal attribute of human nature.

Like medieval tales of knights versus dragons, the literature of the psychotherapeutic case history, dating from Breuer and Freud's *Studies in Hysteria*, typifies one particular epoch. Heroes and fools today parry with the demons of the inner landscape or try to sing them into a docile sleep. The cases that follow are my own contributions to this written tradition. They recount successful psychotherapy with seven people to whom contemporary diagnostic custom would attach a range of labels, from major depression and panic disorder through post-traumatic and dissociative conditions.

Why do I believe these case studies, heirs to so many others, deserve your attention?

First of all, because the cases are real. Each has been read and approved by the patient involved, usually years after the therapy took place. Patients have edited and corrected me, and some have accepted the invitation to have their own reflections included in the text. Disguise and omission has been the minimum possible to maintain privacy without altering the basic stories.

Second is an element of risk. I do my best to welcome surprise and embarrassment, so these cases often lead to unexpected conclusions. As often as not, what I learn does not confirm my initial assumptions (or the patient's). Thus, I have not conquered the psychic landscape in the name of my own theory. I have tried instead to help these people in a practical way.

For these two reasons, I feel satisfied to have held myself to a higher standard than much of the literature, although, like any attempt to describe reality, ours is finally, of course, a "construction."

I call these cases histories "visitations" not because I worked miracles, but because in each of them there was the feeling of being visited—visited by some oblique messenger, usually from the patient's unconscious, whose message ran counter to the patient's (and often my own) conscious process. My role was to listen, to notice, and to amplify sometimes tiny or "insignificant" bits of communication back to the patient himself or herself. If I have a talent, it is that of being able to see the miraculous in what is already there.

Of course there are certain necessary conditions for such visitation to take place. To create them I had to swim against the currents of the psychotherapy profession as it has been evolving in the final decades of the century. While psychotherapy, in general, has become ever more focused and brief, I have taken my time and carried a wide-angle lens. As it has manualized and proceduralized itself, I have kept trying to learn, in Jung's words, "a new language for each patient." And when it has increasingly ignored the Unconscious, I have kept asking for dreams. I couldn't have made the swim on my own; many colleagues have kept faith with this older (but still, after all, quite new) tradition in psychotherapy, providing an alternative consensus within which I could work.

Finally, it should be said that I retell these particular cases because they lend themselves to the telling; they seemed naturally to develop with their own story structures. Overall, the literature of therapy gives an exaggerated impression of its success. Though these seven were successful cases, I assure the reader that I have had many, many failures as well and often learned as much or more from them. Even more important, as far as an accurate depiction of the work is concerned, are the many other successful therapies that simply don't lend themselves well to retelling. A tough slog, after which one may not even have much idea of what went right, is more typical, in my experience, than the exceptional dialogues recounted here.

CASE 1:
DREAM REBUTS THERAPIST

How can it be that psychiatry has abandoned the dream? It is as if Freud and Jung's discovery of an active, unconscious dimension to life has itself been massively repressed! The concept of a parallel and autonomous awareness, with its own "take" on relationships and events, has disappeared into the complicated neural networks with which we now occupy ourselves. We have lost a sense of the forest amid the dendritic trees.

This case illustrates how the simple recognition of the dreamer's Unconscious as a radically separate Other, a third voice in the therapy process, can sometimes save the day. Until it spoke, the patient and I had been busily inventing a new and improved version of his basic problem.

"Dream Rebuts Therapist in a Case of Unresolved Grief" appeared in the February 1995 *Psychiatric Times*.

The general psychiatrist avoids dreams at the patient's peril, as well as his or her own. To adapt once more the old saw about war and generals, dreams are too important to be left to the psychoanalysts—or for that matter to fringe therapists and New Age bookstores. They are a vital, and temporally substantial, part of our life process. When a new resident supervisee recently avowed an interest in learning to work with dreams, my excitement for her was matched by sadness for other new trainees who seem to regard dreams as the quaint preoccupation of a few eccentric historical figures such as Freud and Jung, long superseded by the precise tools of modern medical practice. Not so; they are still the royal road whether we choose to ignore them or not.

It is true that the classic tomes of the old masters are not user-friendly to young people whose education has centered on biology and chemistry rather than history and literature. But these pragmatic psychiatrists may have another more valid suspicion: the complexity of dreams is too easy in which to hide. Working with dreams can be an aesthetically appealing defense mechanism through which patients and therapists avoid dealing directly with each other and with the mundane details of a stalemated life.

Modern dream research and related neuroanatomical studies have indeed disposed of the wish-fulfillment theory in favor of a conception of dream activity as "off-line information processing" (always the computer metaphor) in which problematic situations and affects in current life elicit a search for relevant past experience. Series of dreams in a single night show a personality wrestling with a problem using analogical and metaphorical processes laden with feeling. Sometimes an outsider's interpretive ear in a therapy session can help the patient make fuller use of his own problem-solving capacities by making this unconscious commentary on his life more consciously available; by seizing upon an image or a character as an example of a new possibility for acting or relating to the self or to other people. Such is the art of using dreams.

But to this conventionally practical outlook I find it helpful to add equal parts of awe and respect for the transpersonal wisdom and the danger in that psychic underworld which patients and therapists will never, even in small fraction, understand or illumine or (least of all) control. The dream is our link to that underworld. Its fullest meaning and purpose lies in the dream experience itself and not in the conscious meanings and purposes we impute to it with our dayworld egos.

The case at hand is a particularly useful illustration of this dual view of dreams, in that the patient himself never invested much importance in his dreams or our work with them and tended to forget promptly even those few that we discussed extensively. They did not become a conscious guide or focus for him even though, to me, they artfully encapsulated his ongoing struggle with grief and self-doubt. With two notable exceptions retold below, they were simply core samples from a parallel, unconscious process of personality change, of interest only to me. One of the exceptions, however, represented an intervention by the patient's own unconscious, which was the turning point in the therapy.

He was the kind of man some therapists naturally distrust. Even in clinical depression his handshake was firm and reassuring, complete with purposeful eye contact and a charming smile with a hint of boyish deviltry. The assumed values which underlay his narrative seemed disarmingly innocent: honesty in business and personal life; fair play; marital fidelity; the need to impart a durable morality to one's children; overcoming problems and finding financial success through persistence; systematic but clever thinking; and above all, a positive attitude towards life. In his heyday this success had been mirrored by material circumstance: a boat anchored offshore, popular children, a beautiful wife. There were good friends, good times, and a sense of vital involvement in the commerce of the state.

But when his wife developed a terminal illness it all changed. She railed at him for being a jerk and an asshole (these epithets stung even now, four

years later). His later discovery that she had become addicted to pain medication did not fully assuage his incomprehension of her sudden vindic-
tiveness. Even as he spent most of his savings on heroic last-ditch treatments, she developed a relationship with another man, which ended in
divorce and remarriage only months before her death. As a final insult
from beyond the grave, she had made her wishes known to the children
that she wanted them to leave father for their new stepfather after she was
gone. This they did, depriving my bereft patient of what little solace
might have been left to him.

His life spun aimlessly downward, and for more than a year he had barely
functioned, spending most of his time in bed and haunted by his wife's cries of
"asshole!" which destroyed his self-confidence before he would enter the rare
business meetings he still attempted. If the owner of his company had not also
been a close personal friend, he would have been discarded long since.

In early sessions he sought from me a reinforcement of his own positive-
thinking, up-by-my-bootstraps-and-I'll-get-over-this refrain, which was
patently failing him. After ascertaining that he was far better at these tactics
than me, I opted instead to invite the accusing wife's voice into the room. He
allowed himself to admit that he believed her; that his current shameful failure,
his inability to overcome, only confirmed the truth of her final reproaches.

Attempts at biological treatment followed this same pattern predictably.
His initial reaction was to welcome antidepressants as a potential "jump
start" or "kick in the pants." But his incomplete response to the first agent,
which made it clear that further trials and more prolonged treatment would
be necessary in order to fully exploit that route, compounded his fundamental sense of defectiveness. He decided that he didn't want to "mess with my
mind," that he would "get over this on my own."

The feeling of defect had been lifelong but well-concealed until his
wife's betrayal. Its developmental origins lay in the religious rigidity, moralistic blaming, and emotional distance of his parents, who cultivated a premature autonomy in him and tended to attribute illnesses, injuries, and other
deviations from perfection as signs of personal weakness or lack of resolve.
But my patient had soon discovered gifts which indeed helped him to excel
and "rise above": good looks, verbal facility, and athletic abilities, which even
in his fifties were the envy of men twenty years his junior.

Thus, his best nurturing occurred in the collective, performance-orient-
ed world of sports teams, glee clubs, dramatic societies, and a close-knit fra-
ternity at a high- spirited college. In this world his inadequacies were unwelcome. When he developed a chronic medical condition which forced him to
abandon varsity sports, he shifted to other venues. Ultimately his financial
and social success delivered what school sports had given him earlier on: the
mirror of a sincere and charming man who had his life well in hand.

So having failed very quickly in our efforts at ego support and "de-sham-
ing," the patient and I tried to find the element of truth in his wife's railings

on the therapeutic axiom that such truth would, as it were, set him free from her voice. On the personal level I was ambivalent about this search. I had grown to like and admire this man very much. He was in some ways as different from me as another white male middle-class professional could be. He would ask permission to take the jacket of his three-piece suit off while I slouched in my sweater. On one occasion he regaled me with feats of mnemonics, while I sometimes struggled to remember his or my last sentence. There was a spontaneity about him, even in depression, which my intuition found inconsistent with a "false self" presentation.

I took my misgivings to a peer supervision group. While all took note of the emotional contact I had made with this man and my affection for him, they also emphasized its potential hindrance to a more "objective" investigation of how he had emotionally failed his wife (albeit that her last rantings may have been over-amplified and distorted). True shrinks that we are, we emerged from the meeting with a sense of accomplishment, having once again stood firm together in the therapeutic ship as we steered past the sirens of countertransference. So I returned, re-inoculated with my own belief system and cultural ethos, a societally alienated therapist with a highly developed subjectivity to this all-American patient whom I liked so much.

Christopher Bollas' description of "normotic illness" is a well-elaborated expression of the therapist ethos as it confronts the "antitherapeutic" personality type. Couched in objective diagnostic language, it has nonetheless a damning effect for that which it perceives as opposite to itself:

> "A normotic person is someone who is abnormally normal. He is too stable, secure, comfortable, and socially extraverted. He is fundamentally disinterested in subjective life and he is inclined to reflect on the thingness of objects, on their material reality. Such a person is alive in a world of meaningless plenty.
>
> "... He likes being part of an institution and feels at home in the pseudo-intimacy of teams and committees. This enables him to be identified with the life or the existence of the impersonal: the products of a corporation.
>
> "... He enjoys a good laugh, and seems fun-loving. But rather than experience sadness, he slows down. Friendships are characterized by a mutual chronicling of life's events, rather than by intersubjective exchanges. The capacity to speak frankly about one's own feelings is unknown.
>
> "... There are many rules for right and wrong behavior, but such rules are not really responsive to changing circumstances in life, and do not reflect critical acts of judgement, but obedience to a legalistic introject." [adapted from *The Shadow of the Object*, pp. 137-140.]

If my patient had lived a normotic existence, playing the ideal family man without ever achieving real intimacy with a wife and children who had been fundamentally things in a picture, like the boat, then perhaps the dying, addicted wife's rage and children's desertion made some sense after all. Maybe it had all been a psuedo-life. Our task according to this logic would be to mourn this state of hitherto being "unborn" (in Bollas' words) and to develop a subjective personhood capable of true relationship.

The patient took quickly to such interpretations, advanced piecemeal and with some hesitation on my part. As we both now see, this "normotic" theory was a more sophisticated way of colluding with his own conviction of defectiveness. A richer-sounding verbal formula ("growing subjective personhood") substituted for the "up-by-the-bootstraps" that we therapists find to be in such poor taste. But it was a formula nonetheless, delivered like so many formulas throughout his life had been, from some arbiter of values to my patient, once more labeled defective. If the patient's unconscious had not intervened at this point, we might still be hewing to this pattern today.

Nine months into therapy we obtained the following dream:

The patient is walking at twilight in downtown Portland's brick-paved Monument Square, which appears deserted. A strange rocket or spacecraft noiselessly descends and hovers nearby. It has a transparent nose-cone in which ping-pong balls can be seen bouncing randomly. (His associations revealed that this apparatus had been borrowed from the televised prize-drawings of Northern New England's regional lottery, the infamous "Tri-State Megabucks.") At this moment he hears a terrified woman's scream: his wife's, though she never physically appears. The rocket immediately departs, silently as it had come, leaving my patient, as the only person there, seemingly culpable for a crime he did not commit.

The dream rebutted our defect theory by linking a symbol of random fate—the lottery—with the wife's death, and showing how the patient served as a convenient lightning-rod for her rage at this fate, simply because he was there at the time. We had been unable to see this because her flailing personal attacks were taken in as confirmations of the patient's preexisting sense of defectiveness, which she easily elicited.

The patient then recalled a recent conversation with a childhood friend of his wife's, who had known the wife during her teenage years. During this period the wife's own father had been dying, and the friend told a story of an acquaintance whom the wife had picked out and then systematically and mercilessly tormented over a span of weeks, driving the unfortunate girl to quit their extracurricular school club. So the wife's capacity to divert and focus her rage at fate into pointed cruelty had a history which predated my patient's entry into her life. (This is the kind of insight to which one practicing in a small state is privy.) Her conscious will could act as a magnifying glass, focusing her own experience of nature's random cruelty like the sun's rays as she let it pass through her and burn someone else. Perhaps this capacity to become expressively transparent to the horror one has experienced suggests a definition of individual human evil.

Having been freed by the dream—the gist of which I needed to remind the patient several times in the ensuing weeks, when he would begin reverting to self-blame—we were able to get on with "grief work" in the usual way. Gerald Klerman's "interpersonal" approach, the new academic gold standard in standardized psychodynamic therapies, actually provides a fairly good practical summary of much of what has been learned over the years about working with the bereaved. But the only mention of dreams in the most recent text says that they are not solicited in Klerman's method and, if volunteered by the patient, should be related only to the here-and-now issues. Were I not in the habit of regularly prodding this patient about his dreams, I would not have gotten this dream's message and would have been unable to effectively proceed with the rest of the work Klerman describes.

Four years later the patient wrote, "My sessions with you assisted me in putting some of the bad or guilty feelings in their proper place—namely, behind me, and not inside or on top of me where they were wearing me down twenty-four hours each day. We discussed one dream in particular that helped me learn that my fate had in fact been a random event that was not caused nor controlled by me. That dream was probably the turning point since it came from deep within me, yet was relatively easy to understand and appraise. Thank you for your great assistance."

In a further year of therapy, gradual improvement in energy level and functioning occurred, though never to the previous "driven" level, and therefore never quite fully satisfying to my patient. But he came to see himself as a good but unfortunate man, and eight months after the dream he again permitted a trial of antidepressant, which was helpful this time, not the least because he saw no shame in availing himself of the help. By the time we terminated our regular, by then every other week sessions at twenty-two months, he had deepened a relationship and remarried. The reconciled children and many admiring friends joined in the wedding.

The story of how the ties of fatherhood were mended provided an interesting minor nod to the skepticism of Christopher Bollas. In early letters attempting to register reservations about some of these young people's behaviors (including a habit of using his home as a Maine vacation base without spending time with their father), the patient's tone was distant and moralistic. As therapy progressed his letters shifted from the "you should" to the "you made me feel" tone, and the children were therefore able to hear his anger, pain, and love for them better and had less need to rebel or stay away. So perhaps his subjective realness had needed some deepening after all: a grain of truth in the "normotic" caricature.

A dream near the end of therapy confirmed the inclusiveness of the patient's grieving. Taking his grown children on a pleasant lakeside drive, he by chance encounters his wife, radiantly healthy, walking on the road. They share a passionate kiss, but he does not reverse direction to give her a ride. Having once again experienced the loving contact which had also been a real part of his life with this beautiful and complex woman, he sets off again with the children, going his own way.

CASE 2:
CATFISH ON THE BOTTOM

A companion piece to the last one, this is another instance of the dreamer's Unconscious supplying us with an opposing view to that of the patient herself—one that I seized upon and insistently amplified for her.

This patient's own extensive comments from five years later are the essay's high point. "Catfish" appeared in the December 1995 *Psychiatric Times.*

Consider the nature of a verbal image: It is a word picture which leads beyond words. But it does not bring us into vague emotionality. Rather, it engenders a multimodal experience both highly specific and unique to its hearer. In cognitive/behavioral or hypnotic work, aiming for "relaxation," therapists sometimes enjoin patients to go in their minds, for example, to "a quiet pond." These clinicians have learned that such an image is more effective than simply asking the patient to relax. Why?

To many patients the abstract word "relaxation," or more concrete somatic directives ("take slow, deep breaths"), connote a compliant deadening—in the extreme, an unacceptable surrender of personal autonomy which leads opposite to the desired result. The words' meaning is the property of the therapist. Their instrumental function leads in directions which converge on the therapist's preconceived goals.

The "quiet pond," even in the context of focused therapy, is what has been termed a divergent metaphor, a picture the patient may enter and possess for himself. It may carry peace and tranquility but also has room for the odd ripple, the unseen splash, activity in the dark below the surface. The pond is natural, uncontrolled: its quiet is not coerced. This leaves the patient free to invent his own notion of relaxation that opens into the rest of the patient's life rather than closing him into an externally imposed cure. He is less likely to bolt.

When open-ended, exploratory work is feasible, imagery—particularly patients' own imagery—can truly flourish. This is because its fruits are unpredictable and will not be constrained by time limits, focus, and desired outcomes. Psychiatry more and more emphasizes the latter, often with good reason. But how often is the powerful healing potential latent in imagery thus discarded, unused?

Spontaneous imagery and dreams typically reveal patients' basic assumptions about life, so fundamental and unquestioned as to seem, to the patient, to be simply "the way the world is." Without exception the talented therapists from whom I learned this trade all had the ability to stand such assumptions on their heads at the opportune moments, diffracting patients' imagery through their own personalities, using a critic's ear to help extricate patients from patterns of self-deception.

Here I present a high-achieving woman whose acceptance of self was contingent upon performance. Her highly original, self-invented persona contained much that was true about her. Yet this resourceful and admired individual was blocked from a sense of her own realness. Imagery (here derived from a dream) helped her to develop such a sense, in an unexpected way.

"I'm not thriving," said the striking thirty-year-old engineer, whose specialty was toxicology. She had decided to try therapy because she'd "done everything but." In fact she had probably endured two previous major depressive episodes on her own. Now in a position of relative strength, she characterized her mood as one of "mild despair."

A few years back, emerging from depression, she had shifted her dependence from marijuana to exercise and now worked out three hours per day in addition to studying two different forms of dance. But a tendency to binge eat remained, at once self-soothing and shameful. Relationships with men had been problematic. Her current (and best) one was short on intimacy and long on scheduling. She hesitated to press for the commitment she wanted.

Much about her seemed calculated to impress. In early sessions, her dreams evoked important themes, but were presented as highly structured, almost as works of art. She had read as much contemporary neo-Jungian writing as I had and wove this into the work. Overawed, I felt inarticulate and clumsy in my responses. When I finally used this feeling, remarking on the art-like quality of her persona and my sense of inadequacy before it, she returned next time in shame that I had "found her out" as a forgery.

Indeed, a casual observer would not have guessed that she came from mill-town working class; that both parents were culturally and intellectually limited and mother had spent much of the patient's early childhood in a mental institution; that she had been sexually abused by a relative through her early adolescence. All this she had escaped on the strength of her own gifts: first into the fashion industry and later engineering. So compelling was her aura of sophistication that I found myself wanting to impress her. Once, after the formal close of a session wherein we were beginning to be more comfortable and ordinary with each other—recall the studies that say beginnings and endings are the most telling—I asked her what she thought of a painting I had just purchased. She reverted to her sophisticated self and looked at it intently, chin in hand, before saying a number of complex and articulate things about it.

Next session she returned with dreams of being violated. I realized that I had been drawn into a pattern which was abusive to her. "Why couldn't I have just said, 'It's good' or 'I like it'?" she ruefully asked herself.

Eight months into our weekly sessions she dreamed she had a catfish. From its fishtank she freed it into a pond where it began to grow. When the water drained out, she found a hole in the mud for it. Here it survived until finally the sea rolled in. Now grown large and with a "smile" on its face, it swam away. "I can't believe I'm dreaming about something as ugly as a catfish!" she remarked, seeming disappointed.

"Ugly ... well I don't know. It depends on how you see it. A catfish is beautifully adapted to its environment," I responded.

I reflected aloud to the effect that, her critical intellect notwithstanding, she had been taken in by the New Age, caterpillar-to-butterfly metaphor whereby she would ever transform herself, getting life (and now, therapy) "right" until she became an immortal work of art. Her dream image, which she consciously found repugnant, offered an alternative to this New Age oppression. All she had to do was grow bigger. She has, she is, all she needs from the start. No transformation of her basic nature is required, just freedom, sanctuary, then freedom again.

Although not initially welcomed, this interpretation, or rather inversion of her imagery, opened the way for her to experience the dream's compensatory function. (Though I might have done as well saying a lot less.) She could reconsider the fat, stupid, lost part of herself to which she so feared reverting if she ever relaxed her regime of self-improvement. This "despised self," which heretofore had only appeared in desperation, as a binge eater, contained earthiness, spontaneity, peasant-like strength, and deep wells of a spirituality moving in its simplicity.

The therapy, which lasted two years, was far from over, but the Catfish image became an orienting principle for me to which I would occasionally refer back in sessions. The details of her abuse that she finally entrusted to me involved being shown pornographic magazines in addition to sexual contact. The experience left her with a strong message on "how to be a woman." Without a stable mother to model femininity for her, she was polarized by her adult male abuser into helpless victim and mesmerizing Goddess. This became the template not just for her later pattern of relationships with me and other men but, more generally, for the ceaseless need to be something more. As a man in the sway of this polarity, I became alternately a wielder of arbitrary power and an inept, insecure boy (the latter probably reflecting the way her abuser had felt in the presence of adult women). Falling recurrently into these complementary patterns, we nonetheless struggled at times into real human relationship. I needed to find ways to be forceful without objectifying her; to give her a man's respect. She needed to sort out spontaneity from learned vivaciousness, innate radiance from learned provocativeness.

Going deeper towards the end, we plumbed a core emptiness related to her mother's early failure (she had been institutionalized when the patient was eight months old). My ability to meet the patient in this emptiness was limited, and she was able to become angry at me for that—an opportunity denied her during development. When we finished, the impulse for self-transformation was hardly dead , nor should it have been. But it was better balanced (for me, by the Catfish) with the rest of her that was no longer despised. She felt ready to go on. "I have faith," she insisted.

Five years later, with another depressive episode, she re-entered therapy with a female therapist and, for the first time, started medication treatment. In our contact regarding this paper I invited her to contribute her thoughts and recollections from this distance. She gives the following perspective on our work and the Catfish.

"I recall my distasteful reaction to the Catfish dream when I first shared it in therapy. Notwithstanding that as dreams go it was a pleasant one, at the time my image of the Catfish was hardly positive. For one thing, catfish are bottom dwellers. That is, they tend to live in the lower depths of waterways where it's dark and murky. Second, catfish are not careful eaters; they'll consume whatever's around, including detritus. They are also lipophilic (literally fat-loving) and tend to retain environmental toxins. Thus they are among the most contaminated members of the ecosystem. And then, of course, they are ugly.

"For these reasons I would have been content with simply reporting my dream (as I had become accustomed to doing in our therapy sessions) and going on to something else more compelling. I think I found my therapist's reaction to the Catfish dream irritating. I felt like he was trying to sell me on ordinariness. My unspoken response to that was 'Thanks but no thanks.'

"Since the time of that dream and associated therapy, I have gained more of an appreciation for catfish. Catfish are survivors. For example, some can walk (albeit ungracefully) out of the water and onto land, if need be. Other species, during times of stress (such as cold temperatures or extreme chemical toxicity), are able to bury themselves in the mud until conditions improve. I also learned that although catfish don't grow well in small ponds, if they can find their way to larger water bodies, they tend to thrive.

"Depression can make you feel like you're in the mud. Though it can be a form of refuge, there is the fear of being stuck there forever, alone in the dark, cold, surrounded by contamination. Even if you manage to emerge, there is a sense of dread at the thought of returning. So, you try hard not to go back. I tried many ways not to go back. When something I tried seemed to help, I went for more and more of it. My survival techniques became addictions. Eventually though, I would wind up back in the mud. And so it goes.

"It takes a tremendous amount of energy to maintain the cycle of extremes. I went to therapy mostly out of exhaustion. I was tired of frantically swimming back and forth in the same small pond. I think one important thing that therapy has helped me to do is to go back into the mud, but in a safer way. It's given me the opportunity to be there, to feel it, to look at it, and to see what's pure and what's poison, with the reassurance of a compassionate and able hand to hold onto if I need help getting back. In this way I have been able to feed on the nourishment of its rich organic matter, and this has helped me to grow. Over time I have learned that I can swim—freely, slowly, and with a smile."

For me, one of the most enjoyable duties of the analytic therapist is the need to remain skeptical of prevailing cultural wisdom. In our time, that wisdom is itself therapeutic. I believe the Catfish image helped free this patient from her New Age transformative prison. Through the course of our work, the image could hang like a knitter's loose end from the fabric of the therapy, ready to be picked up and knitted in when it became necessary to remind the patient of a different way of seeing herself, in the language of her own unconscious. She learned that what is complex and artful may nevertheless be wrong; that sometimes, humble platitudes speak the truth. "I am what I am and that's all that I am" (to quote Popeye's song) moves, in the patient's written recollection, from a confining "ordinariness" to a unique, bottom-dwelling survivorship rooted in her personal history.

I am no student of aboriginal religions, but all of them of which I am aware ascribe special import to the spirits of animals. From the Native American "stray" to the Australian "walkabout," individuals search for an animal which is a sign—which has a special personal meaning for them. The totem animal's qualities present a living example which calls something forth, something that is unique and intrinsic to the human seeker. It seems fitting, in an age where we live cut off from a de-spirited nature, that the Catfish would have to swim to my patient from a dream. But these totems may equally well show themselves to us in the daytime as we hurry across some fragmentary patch of green.

Though she moved on to new images, insights, and central concerns, the Catfish remains this patient's totem in my own memory of her: a creature whose form captured something palpable and naively vital in this outwardly accomplished and sophisticated woman.

CASE 3:
THE PERMANENT TRIP

Here is a situation where an experiential risk paid off. I have never seen the visual world in quite the same way since. One could say that the intervention here was primarily cognitive—and I'm no snob about that—but I would argue that it was equally important that I joined the patient in his isolated perceptual world as a companion.

"Trip" first came out in the Winter 1995 issue of *Voices*; it was reprinted, with a commentary by the biological psychiatrist Ronald Pies, in April 1998's *Psychiatric Times*, subtitled with the new nomenclature for the problem: "Hallucinogen Persisting Perception Disorder." Pies' scientific observations were greatly appreciated, but seemed too specialized to include in this version.

Dan, twenty-one, was home from college in the middle of the winter, having dropped out after a miserable year and a half. His problems had begun about three years before, shortly after period of drug experimentation which had included three LSD trips. A few weeks after his final trip, newly abroad as an exchange student, he began experiencing spontaneous visual hallucinations including moving "dots" in the visual field, afterimages or "blurs" of moving objects, a sense of being able to "see the air," and other phenomena described by Abraham (1983; see also DSM-IV, pp.233-4) as "post-hallucinogen perception disorder." Neither his hosts nor the European physicians he eventually saw had any clue about what was wrong, and Dan sensed they were beginning to think he was a hypochondriac, so he stopped complaining and endured this problem on his own for a year, fearing for his sanity. Not until he started college back in the U.S. did he find his way to a neurologist and eventually to Abraham himself, who made the definitive diagnosis and found "persistent activation of the right posterior temporal area" after visual evoked response testing. [The electrical activity in the brain's visual cortex, generated in response to a test stimulus, did not die away within the expected amount of time but kept on going for much longer.]

The symptoms were managed with clonazepam [trade name Klonopin, a potent relative of the familiar Valium] on the theory that their neurologic basis might resemble siezure activity. Dan seemed to require high and ever-increasing dosages and became withdrawn and depressed. He stopped functioning in school and socially, drank alcohol more heavily, and when he realized what was happening to him, finally decided to come home.

My suspicion when I began working with Dan was that the clonazepam was a major contributor to his depression. But my initial efforts to taper the dose, while working in conventional psychotherapy on developmental issues behind his sense of being punished by his perceptual affliction, met with resistance and a florid worsening of the visual symptoms. Then, four months into the work, came the session when I spontaneously sat next to him on the couch, looking out the office window at a clear blue sky, and asked him to describe what he saw. As he began I tried to "suspend" my habitual state of consciousness and see whether any of his "hallucinations" were visible to me. To my surprise, I was immediately able to see irregular linear shapes floating slowly across the visual field. When I blinked, they would change shape or position. I began describing this to Dan in great detail so he would have no doubt that I was not simply repeating his descriptions but actually having my own similar experiences. Clearly these "shooters" seemed to be generated by something on the surface of the eye to which we don't normally attend. I invite the reader to try this for him/herself.

In this and a few succeeding sessions I was able to experience *with Dan* most of the phenomena of his illness, including visual "trails" of moving objects; various line-shape illusions, such as level bookshelves slanting; "aeropsia," a sense of bright whiteness in the air between us and observed objects; and "dancing bright spots" originating between the letters and words on a printed page. With minimal information from him I could describe these convincingly, at times even completing his sentences. We both found this a strangely exhilarating activity. It was clear to me, however, that I did not experience these visual phenomena as intensely and persistently as did he and that I could ignore them at will.

Whatever the physiological mechanism of this disorder may be, it is obvious that functionally a failure of a normal preconscious "editing" process was occurring, whereby additional irrelevant aspects of raw perceptual experience were reaching consciousness.

Dan reported a great sense of relief and "normalization" as a result of these few sessions. Tapering down his clonazepam to a very minimal dosage was now accomplished with relative ease. Predictably, the major depressive symptoms resolved. There was much else to talk about in a year of therapy, but we both agreed, and still agree several years later, that our perceptual experiment was the turning point.

Before our mutual experiences, the symptoms "meant" that Dan was crazy, different from other people, alone forever in a distorted visual universe. This triggered a vicious cycle, or "positive feedback loop," in which Dan's anxiety about this situation served to amplify the symptoms in his conscious awareness and continually refocus his attention upon them. Thus the ordinary distractions of everyday experience were unable to perform their potentially useful role, powerless to divert him from an "illness" which became the center of his life, and expectably, a crystal nidus for fantasies of punishment which sprang from their usual developmental lairs. He was quite capable of understanding the sources of this hitherto-latent shame, but this did not impact his perceptual distortions one whit.

After the "normalization," though, Dan had only the symptoms themselves with which to contend and not the snowballing anxiety and sense of retribution. He became more distractible in the healthy sense, his conscious attention freer to roam or focus elsewhere (studies, relationships). And through the experience (and perhaps, I'll allow, as a result of our developmental work as well—sudden "miracles" usually have some amount of groundwork preceding them) he had found his way to a more thoroughgoing self-acceptance.

Dan returned to a different college, did very well, and got his degree. He now works in the mental health field. For the past seven years the same low dose of clonazepam has been necessary, but with it, except in times of extreme stress or physical fatigue, he is rarely bothered by visual symptoms.

CASE 4:
LACAN AT BONUS BAGELS

Some of my regular readers from the *Psychiatric Times* found this piece to be "out of character" for me. I have often played the down-home, country psychiatrist in my column there, and here I was spouting trendy Parisian theories in a somewhat different tone. In fact, this patient brought me directly to the tension within myself between the Ivy-educated intellectual and the provincial rustic. It took the appearance of a better integrated figure in his dream to lead both of us out of this hamstrung position.

"Lacan" appeared in the May 1998 *Times*.

Working with the intellectually gifted is not as easy as one might think. With all that conceptual ability, patients like the young man I am about to describe—whose basic predicament could equally well occur in the life of a high-school dropout—can get quite literally "way ahead of themselves." Such patients can think and verbalize far beyond their level of emotional development. In my experience, well-grounded therapists with few intellectual pretensions are often the best choice for these brilliant people. They provide something simple, honest, and direct, "cutting through the bullshit" to the human being whose essence is just like any other.

For me, a dilettante in love with words and ideas, there is the risk of missing what the patient really needs from therapy. It can be such a joy to play with allusions and concepts (akin to meeting someone who speaks one's native language in a roomful of foreigners) that wordplay may be all that happens, and inarticulate pain may be left untouched. Or the play can turn less mutual, into a sort of covert competition. In the six months this case gave us together, each of these pitfalls took its turn. But if Robert Bly is right that a major cultural task of older men is to admire younger men who are not their sons, I at least felt equipped to admire this wonderfully literate and talented person.

20

At our best, we could collaborate in achieving a lightly ironic tone whose humor left room for the painful aspects of this man's situation to be fairly expressed. Thus, in an early session, he described his habit of reading alone at a table in a coffee shop, behind a stack of books, wanting but not wanting contact. In the authors—Foucault, Lacan, Derrida—he found voices passionately subversive to the falseness, the dehumanizing commodification of the social world in which we are all immersed. Yet the display of books itself could not escape a function within that world, as he readily agreed. These icons of the postmodern, deconstructionist intellectual scene were placed to attract. They said to the passerby (preferably young and female, but really, anyone who cared), in effect, here sits an interesting person, someone you want to know. More concretely, the books were physical barriers behind or within which an anxious young man could hide.

His episodic anxiety attacks had begun in his first semester of graduate school. He didn't know what he wanted. In absentia, his love for a girlfriend left behind in a distant city grew deeper; he composed poetry for her as he wandered along littered railroad tracks. But when she readied herself to move to him, he found himself panicking. He was at a loss to explain his doubts in painful long-distance conversations with her. Looking back on it from my office, he realized that he found her single-minded focus on him, her "lack of other interests," disturbing.

Although he had quickly made an impression as the class Lacan expert in his prestigious humanities doctoral program, he couldn't concentrate well enough to put his thoughts on paper for coursework. He called home in tears. His parents' support and understanding was exemplary, but they had conflicting takes on his situation. Mother encouraged him to take his questioning seriously. Father, reasoning soberly about all the ways in which this young couple was compatible, favored a clear-eyed commitment.

He never finished the fall's papers. Driving to the girlfriend's, he felt trapped and "hysterical" upon arriving at her empty apartment. She returned and they spent a tense, inconclusive weekend. He went back to the family home, telling his professors that he needed time to sort things out. A leave of absence was arranged; his work was promising and he would be welcome back next year. So he came to me and to the table at Bonus Bagels and started looking for a job.

We started—as, I ventured, Lacan might—with what the patient was not talking about. Despite his gifts, he was not immune from dependent longings, a need for security in a suddenly vast adult world. He doubted his ability to sustain himself independently, as anyone would if willing to admit it. So the press in his love poems told me little about who his girlfriend was and much about his need for a feminine presence to see and treasure him in a world which imperiled his uniqueness. To simply label this by one of its instinctual sources—needing Mother—was wrong and reductive but crudely necessary in order to separate the story of two young people from the internal drama of his own conflicting needs.

For if he needed emotional safety to flower, he also needed room. The trapped panic betrayed his doubts about whether this particular person, befriended so early in life, would be able to afford him such room. His dreams illustrated both sides of this "near/far dilemma" in colorful ways. Through them, through his poetry, and much conceptualizing on both our parts we arrived quite richly at a prosaic conclusion: He wasn't yet ready to make this kind of commitment.

If he was learning anything cognitive from me, it was to think more consciously in polarities like this instead of being unconsciously buffeted by them, as is the perennial human habit. As he stepped back from his relationship and surveyed his life and his family of origin, he relaxed a bit in sessions, becoming less anxious and less relentlessly articulate. The outlines of the "regular guy" his father had initially described to me became visible alongside his brilliance.

But as he tried to complete his coursework, a persistent writer's block demonstrated that there must have been more than desperate indecision about his woman friend that had hung him up the past fall. His outwardly polished academic persona was running into another set of obstacles. He had clearly impressed his professors (and me), but he just plain hadn't lived long enough to have read everything, so whenever he came to a provisional conclusion or a plausible argument, there was always another point of view to consider, another classic author to digest. He wanted, in these graduate-school term papers, to be nothing less than final and definitive! And so he couldn't write. He wondered whether he should do something else with his life.

Here is one point where my expensive education probably helped me with this patient. If I learned anything at Harvard, it was how to appear as if I know and have read much more than I do or have. I could therefore appreciate the magnitude of the socialization process bearing down on this young man. This process is all the more ironic when it emanates from critical academia, a marvelously competitive hierarchy which claims to subvert what in fact it perpetuates. But as usual it took the patient's own unconscious to find a way out of this latest near/far dilemma: "definitive," imitative security versus inarticulate failure.

The Unconscious cast my patient in a dream as the pop singer Michael Jackson. The music star's well-publicized quest for eternal boyhood in both attitude and appearance (Jungians call him a *puer* figure) contrasted with what he was trying to do: play NBA basketball with the Chicago Bulls. While pop stars these athletes may also be, the patient's sense of danger and of fraudulence seemed to emphasize that another African-American Michael, Michael Jordan, and his crew, were initiated men playing a man's game for keeps. My patient did not belong out there.

Realizing this, the "authorities" had him ejected from the game, arrested, and sent off to jail. Enroute he was visited by a friend from work (in waking life, the patient had found a lawn care job for the season). Knowing that my patient, who by now had resumed his usual appearance, was to be imprisoned, this young friend from Al's Landscaping had brought a gift to help him sustain himself there.

The "Al's Landscaping guy," as we were to name this figure afterward, was typical of a few of the men my patient had befriended on the job: slightly older; sharp but unschooled; witty; and possessed of good common sense. Standing there in his work clothes he offered the patient a book—not Habermas, not Rilke, but a tattered old high school American history text. It was, no doubt, an oversimplified "secondary source." It did not glitter with deconstructionist theory. But it was obviously well thumbed and well loved by the friend. The Al's Landscaping guy offered, as solace, a book that had meant something to him; that he had made a part of himself.

So here was an image of the patient's True Self. He was indeed a "regular guy," but one who loved ideas, even ideas that were not fashionably dressed. Speaking in his own words about his own ideas was more than a resolution to the academic near/far dilemma. It was, in fact, the only way to survive in prison—the "iron cage" of isolated existence in a society which tends to objectify and commodify its members.

As work with dreams like this one began to free up the patient's ability to write, it turned out that the content of his major paper, like that of the dreams themselves, derived directly from his struggle for authentic identity. He was fascinated by the drawings of an artist who worked with his eyes closed, attempting pointedly thereby to frustrate the viewer's preconceptions about what his drawings "represented" or of who he, the artist, was and what he might be "saying" in the drawing. To this artist my patient applied the psychoanalytic concepts of Jacques Lacan.

Mirrors for Lacan are not the nurturing selfobjects of Kohut. Lacan's "mirror stage," though placed with scientific-sounding precision by the French theorist between six and eighteen months of age, seems best taken as an alternative developmental metaphor—the more so when one considers that some historical cultures have not had mirrors for their infants to gaze into. The idea from *Ecrits* (which I hastened to read) goes like this. The infant at this stage—clumsy, largely helpless, and filled with inchoate sensations and instinctual desires—is not an integrated being but only a "becoming." But on seeing itself reflected back in the mirror, a premature identification with a spatial whole, an "I," occurs. Thereafter, this misrecognition (*méconnaissance* = mis-knowing) of self as an ideal and capable person leads "to the assumption of the armor of an alienating identity, which will mark with its rigid structure the subject's entire mental development." The growing individual, cut off from the unintegrated but living reality of his actual emotional maturation, strives instead to mimic the integrated image whose very completion, for a developing child, is a kind of death.

This false and restricting sense of self derived from an external image will, according to Lacan, be further elaborated by the messages of language

23

and culture that ceaselessly tell us who and what we are throughout life. Thus Lacan's persistent popularity among social theorists and literary critics: His "mirror stage," whether literally true of child development or not, provides a retrospective myth about childhood which makes a compelling statement about the adult self embedded in modern consumer culture.

And so at this critical juncture in his life, my patient had been caught between two mirrors. An incompletely educated, emotionally still developing young man, he was being rushed into the image of a committed, monogamous spouse on the one hand, and/or an erudite Lacanian academic on the other. Even Lacan's verbal analysis couldn't save him from these mirrors since Lacan's intellectuality could itself equally become a mirror of definitive formulations and unassailable arguments which would undermine the wide-open, youthful searching he had ahead of him. His anxiety symptoms, in forcing him to back off from everything and temporarily, at least, withdraw from school and relationship, proved to be his only salvation (and what a waste it would have been to medicate away this vital signal!). Like his artist subject, he had, in effect, closed his eyes in order to elude suffocation by the preconceptions of the culture.

As the therapy wound down the patient, no longer anxious, developed a new kind of confidence. This was not the pressured, imitative confidence of the "I" in Lacan's mirror, but a more cautious attitude well aware of his own vulnerability. He was ready to remain as yet unformed and to resist those seductive social contexts which would seek to define his becoming prematurely as being—most particularly, that literate academic world which he was re-entering and within which he had such potential to thrive.

If we had been able to work long term—and in truth, I don't feel that this would necessarily have been a good thing, offering, as therapy does, another seductive mirror—I might have accomplished two further things. First, I might have better answered the question we both had about the origins of his exquisite sensitivity to the modern condition as incarnated in his particular "girl and school problems." The patient was a handsome and socially attractive man whose talents extended beyond academics to the athletic and the artistic. Was his simply a temperamental sensitivity, or had his experience in the family of origin somehow cultivated his perceptiveness? And second, I might have had the pleasure of simply sitting—sweating, breathing, and inarticulate—as a middle-aged man with a younger man. Such intimacy only rarely leaked around the seal of the professor/student archetype.

At two year's distance, the patient, now happily back at graduate school, offers a description of how his dream friend influenced the next phase of his life:

"Upon returning to graduate school the year before last, I made an effort to find a balance between my work and those activities that had always been a part of my life before committing to academics. But joining a soccer team, playing my drums (without too many complaints from my neighbors) and having more of a social life were not the only things that helped me work through what I had spent several months discussing in therapy. I found that my reflections on a few key dreams were finding their way into discussions with friends about our emotional lives in graduate school. I saw the significance of figures such as the man from 'Al's Landscaping' come alive when I was engaged in conversation, not from retelling the dream, but from finding simple words to match the emotional quality of its imagery. These conversations made me feel that I was sharing a story about my experience, registering both its uniqueness and its universality. In this way, I think I have continued to benefit from the images and scenarios in which I had cast my encounters with anxiety."

This engagement with the intellect of a young cultural critic forces me to question myself in inconvenient ways. In writing about him am I commodifying his story for my own narcissistic ends? Imprisoned as I am by the same social forces as he, am I not at this moment making a display so as to appear interesting, attractive, someone you want to know? And at the same time, safe behind the barrier of my articulate case history?

The affirmative answer is obvious. But nonetheless, the patient and I agree that the man from Al's Landscaping deserves to be heard by more than just the two of us. We want the work-suited gardener with the heartfelt gift to instruct us all as we find our ways through the hall of mirrors that is contemporary social life.

CASE 5:
LIVING WITH DOUBT

In the late 1980s in the U.S., a collective hysteria possessed the psychotherapy community. Childhood sexual abuse (depressingly common as it is), usually "repressed," was irresponsibly invoked as an explanation for just about everything. Respected authorities spoke seriously about having patients with "95 alter personalities," and specialized inpatient units arose for the treatment of "Satanic Cult Abuse."

My own entries into the Recovered Memory controversy tried to thread a needle between reactive denial, on the one hand, and the prevailing trends which divided people and their families further and insisted on absolute "belief" on the therapist's part. My viewpoint did not fit easily into either polarized camp, and so I was only able to publish my writing on the subject much later, after better-known people had begun to publicly question the situation.

This case finally appeared in *Psychiatric Times* in November 1996. Trauma-oriented treatment has moved on since this therapy took place, but I include "Doubt" here because its lessons transcend the historical controversy about Recovered Memory. In their applicability to long-term therapy in general, they have stood the test of time.

This patient, too, made interesting and extensive comments several years later.

If I am ever blessed with the time to reflect back on my career as a therapist, a handful of cases will stand out like signposts along the road. I present this one because the four years since its completion have served, if anything, to increase its relevance to a number of the ongoing controversies in our field. Most obvious of these is the "Recovered Memory" debate of which I wrote in an earlier paper ["Reality by Decree," *Psychiatric Times*, November 1993—not included in this collection]. But what I learned from this patient transcends that debate, having become an underpinning of my own views on the nature of, and rationale for, long-term psychotherapy in general. The case is thus especially important for me to remember in this era when biological and/or short-term paradigms have come to dominate psychiatric practice.

Imagine, if you will, the kind of unhurried termination which was routinely possible in the mid-1980s. I have successfully treated this thirty-year-old woman with post-partum depression over about a year, having begun our work several months after the birth of her first child. When we started she had already discontinued the tricyclic antidepressant her obstetrician had prescribed, which had been of definite but limited benefit. [Tricyclics were the standard antidepressant medications before the better-tolerated Prozac and its heirs largely supplanted them in the 1990s.]

Clearly still quite depressed and tearful at first, she had gradually improved without medication as she allowed herself, provisionally, to express her pain and ask for help with a little less shame. Her mother had had a psychotic episode in the patient's youth which had stigmatized her in their small town. At all costs my patient did not want to be "crazy like my mother," as getting psychiatric help initially implied. I still recall how mortified the patient was when I helped push her car out of a snowbank one afternoon after a session—one of the gifts "real life" occasionally gives to the therapeutic process. By the end, her intense shame had yielded to an irritated embarrassment, and she was glad to feel like she didn't need me anymore. She still appeared to lack a sense of herself as a good and deserving person and to be rigid in style, but her momentum was leading her away from my office. I didn't presume to fight it.

But there would be one jarring event that made my concern for her future less theoretical. In one of our last sessions she anxiously related how she had just succumbed to what she called a "telephone rape." A man had called claiming to be a college student doing research on womens' clothing preferences. By the end of the "interview" with this ingratiating psychopath, my patient had been induced through a cleverly incremental series of questions and invitations to masturbate while on the phone. Her tale of this humiliation (I was glad she would trust me with it) revealed a vulnerable aspect of which I had been completely unaware. She most definitely did not want to change her termination plans on its account, however. She only wanted me to know about it. I did not disguise my misgivings, but we agreed it would remain a loose end.

She returned about a year later, six days post-partum from child number two and severely depressed. This time we both agreed that rapid biological control was called for and were able to establish it with another tricyclic. But the medication could not erase her sense of having "failed" a second time, and a host of incoherent emotions emerged: She felt guilty for some unspecifiable horrid, aggressive act, then enraged at having been "falsely accused." I could make no sense of it. Concluding after a few sessions that therapy was "causing more problems than it solves," she opted for medication treatment only.

Three months later she was back, indecisive, anhedonic, wishing she were dead, and at last willing to settle in. I titrated the antidepressant by blood level, and reasoning that her mother's psychotic illness may have been bipolar, augmented with lithium within a few weeks when her depression proved resistant [again, standard psychiatric practice]. In another few weeks, with symptomatic control tenuously re-established, the "alter" or split-off personality fragment made its debut.

First appearing during a therapy session, this frightening "gargoyle" or monster also had a small-child quality. It was hitting and shooting a gun at my patient, yelling "_____ must die!" Able to see all of this with eyes open and me simultaneously in sight, the patient described these goings-on to me. No negotiation was possible, but when the monster's fury seemed to have spent itself, my patient made an instinctive, spontaneous response, which to me still epitomizes why she eventually came through this therapy successfully. In her visualization, she held her tormentor in her arms. She would not always be able to maintain such compassion in the face of savage attacks.

A dam had burst, and we were occupied for the better part of a year in keeping ourselves afloat amidst a flood of such material, in and out of sessions. Typically, she would narrate visually experienced scenes featuring her interacting wordlessly with the alter. The alter never spoke through the patient to me, nor did other personalities appear—but then, I never persistently invited such phenomena of her. If I had, I wonder whether I might have uncovered (or perhaps, precipitated) a more classical "multiple personality" presentation.

The patient was so highly dissociable in the therapy context that at times she was reluctant to sit down at the beginning of a session. Formal hypnotic inductions were never necessary, though she would sometimes close her eyes to focus exclusively on her internal experiences. Frequent vivid dreams and more rarely voices inviting suicide amplified her experience of "falling apart." Sometimes I needed to remind the alter, through the patient, that if it killed her it might never get to tell its story. But along with the patient's desperation and deteriorated functioning came a visible increase in vitality. Her movements were more fluid, her voice more inflected as time went on.

The first suggestions that the patient may have had sexual contact with her father were indirect, just vague feelings of dread, and occurred a couple of months into the "gargoyle" phase. Within a few sessions incestuous imagery (at first symbolic, then more graphic) had entered the dissociative visual experiences she would have in the office. At one point she dreamed of making an incision in her abdomen and aborting a new life inside her, the idea of incest with her "good" parent being so threatening. As if to reply, the monster brutally stabbed her during a spontaneous dissociation. It would not be aborted.

28

The year was 1989, and the popular fascination with sexual abuse was at its height. It was hard to avoid becoming convinced, as I did, that this patient too had been a victim. In my defense, I will say that I did my best not to force this conclusion upon the patient (who, incidentally, had not saturated herself in advance with the "incest survivor" literature). It would have been equally dishonest not to share my thinking with her. The idea of a personality split originating in abuse would explain why this compliant, depressive individual hadn't been able to marshal enough anger to defend herself against the telephone voyeurist, for example. It would make eminent sense that, given her intrusive, psychotic mother, the patient had a dire need to preserve at least one adequate parent. A dissociative split could accomplish this, leaving her "primary personality" free to idealize the actually somewhat distant and unreliable father. Consultation with a specialist colleague seemed to confirm my suspicions, but could, of course, prove nothing. Meanwhile, the child-monster evolved into a more benign figure which the patient called "the Five-Year-Old." Over many more months this figure acted as a "guide" to further visualized scenes of incest, in many of which the father's physical form was grotesquely distorted.

About a year after these intense dissociative experiences had begun, evidence about the nature of the patient's emotional disturbance emerged from another quarter: outward life. Her work supervisor, going through a divorce, became depressed and began confiding in her. Though not attracted to this man, my patient felt a strong "duty" to offer herself to him sexually, in the hopes of somehow healing him. The urge became strong enough and the fantasy detailed enough that she was forced at one point to call her husband at home to prevent herself from going out after work with this confused man, whose boundaries appeared to be all too weak.

This episode was a turning point in the therapy because it provided a present-day reality within which the patient could explore her misbegotten sense of "duty" and begin to set a new kind of boundary for herself: all without having to decide on the "yes or no" of theorized past incest.

Boundaries became, in this next phase, the order of the day. The Five-Year-Old, while never exactly cooperative, became an (at times, playful) collaborator. In dreams and spontaneous trance the alter's focus shifted from relentless scenes of incest to reactions to current relationships with supervisor, husband, myself. The Five-Year-Old's reactions were often dramatically different from the patient's own conscious responses: rage at someone's unreasonable demand versus her conscious guilt over having failed to fulfill it, for example. Paradoxically, the alter's "commentaries" sometimes registered fear at some newly assertive action taken by the patient herself, as if she had gone too far, too fast for the alter's own liking.

I won't pretend that it was clear sailing from here, but in retrospect, such negotiated three-way dialogue increasingly typified the second half of this four-year therapy. (I should mention here that medications were easily tapered and discontinued about halfway through without recurrence of major affective symptoms.)

One context within which a boundary against violation-masquerading-as-duty needed to be set was particularly ironic: an incest survivors' therapy group. I had referred the patient to such a group, run by the therapist colleague I had consulted with before; she began attending shortly after the supervisor episode. Although "certainty" on the patient's part was not required, both the therapist and the other group members seemed to act as if my patient's ultimate belief in a past experience of incest was inevitable. She felt patronized by these women and dreamed of them all sitting at little desks in a grade-school class taught by the therapist. After several attempts to address this feeling within the group failed, she left it, with my support. The group had indeed "accelerated her process," but in a way quite different than I or its leader had envisioned. This patient would not be violated by the certainty of others.

Eventually the patient needed to have me make an official, explicit statement about my goals for her *vis à vis* the "truth" of her incest imagery and the need for "fusion" with her Five-Year-Old alter. Letting her continue to heal far outweighed any theoretical agenda. To impose a textbook resolution upon her would be to violate her again—to become one more powerful figure (supposedly more benign) who would decree what her reality should be. I told her that having her be "sure" about incest or fusing her with the Five-Year-Old were not prerequisites for our work as far as I was concerned. Her dual reaction was as follows. The conscious self, relieved, took this as a statement that we were done and wanted to leave. The Five-Year-Old felt abandoned, that I was uninterested; she clearly wanted to be with me longer.

The admixture (not fusion) of these two reactions informed the lengthy final phase of the therapy, as the patient consciously explored her frustrations in having a relationship with me within the transference. Initially caught between the poles of too-rigid boundaries or no boundaries at all, she reinvented the wheel, or the "semi-permeable membrane" (an image we drew from her own scientific background). By the time we were through she had probed my limits, experiencing first-person affection, rage, and flirtatiousness with me while coming to recognize that perfect safety, even here, was a dangerous illusion. The Five-Year-Old's dissociative appearances became less frequent but her status as an independent whistle blower was maintained. Dreams ranged further afield. At termination, one cogently summed up what we had achieved. The patient was going on a trip and had somehow forgotten her baggage. But she was wearing a new leather jacket, emblematic, I felt, of a tough but flexible "skin" or boundary.

This being a small state, I have seen or heard from this patient with some regularity in the four years since [and now it is ten years], and I interviewed her on the occasion of this paper. She continues to do well and takes no psychoactive medication; the Five-Year-Old appears only rarely, in times of stress.

Open-ended, long-term psychotherapy is being rapidly discarded by psychiatry's mainstream in the late 1990s. Yet I cannot help feeling that its application in the case of this remarkable person (as well as many others whose stories remain unwritten) was in some sense definitive. I don't pretend to any certainty that it will provide ironclad prophylaxis against future affective episodes. With 1990s eyes I am quite aware of her bipolar vulnerability and recall vividly a few brief periods of over-energized, pressured elation. But if she ever should have the misfortune of becoming psychiatrically ill again I am sure that she would face her condition as a far stronger, better integrated individual, and thus expect its treatment would be simpler. At this point she has had, at least, far less exposure to maintenance medication than she would have if I had mistaken the Five-Year-Old's relentless purposiveness for a psychotic symptom.

This was a woman who needed me to throw away the books. Externally imposed truth, whether in the form of the then-contemporary insistence on the "fact" of incest and on fusion or in the guise of today's short-term manuals, would not have served her well. She had to explore her inner world in her own way and time, or not at all.

Quite apart from this patient's dissociative imagery depicting incest, the circumstantial evidence of the "telephone rape" and the work supervisor episode still seem quite compelling suggestions of it. But in the end, we may never know whether literal, physically realized incest ever happened to her—or need to. In this regard she tells me that, had she settled near her parents, more of a "decision" may have been necessary for her. But she didn't, and she enjoys her infrequent visits with her father when they occur.

So she lives with doubt, and this is what she has taught me to do. Toward the end of our work, she became active in jazz dance. The studio provided a safe place for her to discover anew her physicality and sexuality. I never saw her dance, but if I picture her leaping with joy and a hint of fear, I can have an image of the life-giving force that a willingness to live with doubt can free.

The patient wrote these thoughts at four years distance. [She remains well ten years on.]

"If therapy hadn't been long term, I don't know if the Five-Year-Old would have appeared. I may have flitted from therapist to therapist trying to get to the cause but never feeling safe enough to expose her. If she had appeared and then my allotment of sessions ran out, I would have been suspended in a horrible state. And so I am thankful for the opportunity to 'do my work' just the way it was done.

"During those years, my mind was preoccupied with her stuff. My evaluations at work were the lowest ever. I was told that people didn't know how to talk to me, that I was unpredictable. I simply couldn't keep my mind on much of anything. Though I love to read, I don't think there is a single book that I read for pleasure during that time.

"The Five-Year-Old still exists. I don't interact with her often, but I couldn't destroy her any more than I could destroy a physical friend who had helped me through a hard time. She doesn't run my life, but accents it, and helps me when I'm confused about things. Writing this up, I thought I would try to contact her. She was in a good mood to start with, but then seemed frustrated and angry. She didn't think I appreciated how difficult her job was. Anyways, she said 'It is too hard, I can't keep it all straight.' She then opened a catch-all drawer—that drawer in the kitchen that is never organized. It has the odd spatulas, the vegetable peeler, etc., tossed into it. The drawer was overflowing. It was a bit humorous. We shut the drawer together, agreeing that 'It doesn't matter anyway.'"

CASE 6:
"I'M NOT YOUR URBAN
RENEWAL PROJECT"

My good friend, the Atlanta psychologist Margaret Nichols, has observed that sometimes patients will arrive in her practice and she'll just want "to sit at their feet and learn." This was one such case. I don't necessarily recommend trusting one's spontaneous responses as a general rule, but there are some remarkable people one encounters for whom doing anything else seems wrong.

In previous essays I have described dream figures that appear to compensate for an imbalance in the conscious view. It is as if this patient herself was such a figure for me, calling much of what I thought I knew about trauma and its treatment into question

"Urban Renewal" appeared in the February 2000 *Psychiatric Times*.

Over the years a handful of our most gifted clinician/theorists, D.W. Winnicott and Leston Havens among them, have complained that psychiatry has never convincingly described emotional health—excepting, of course, as the *absence* of the various pathologies on which we have been so articulate. At work in my own office I often fumble with patients' questions about what is "normal," succeeding only in separating out the idea of average from a more elusive concept of "optimal." My recognition of health has never been systematic. It has been built up from fragmentary experiences of patients' lives. I have learned mostly to congratulate and support what I recognize.

Nowhere have I witnessed thriving psychological health more clearly than in the life of an African-American woman, now in her thirties, whose therapist I happened to become during a transition year between school and the beginning of her professional career. Mind you, none of the elements of health that I recognized in this patient is unique to her. She would be the first to assert that she is not a saint; like all of us, she remains capable of human

33

cruelty and all the other sins. The outcome of whatever further tests may lie ahead for her remains unknown. If we allow, as I do, that she is a sort of heroine, she must not as such represent just her own race or gender. Her most severe challenges were universal ones.

I prefer to avoid idealization by describing health not as a person but as a *response* to the challenge of the human condition. Here I will attempt to describe the health that one articulate patient demonstrated—or rather embodied—at just a few selected junctures in her life history and in her hours with me. My thoughts yield at times to the temptation to *explain why*, but my goal is only to *describe how*; to center on a phenomenology of health. Unlike Havens or Winnicott, I will be happy if my bearing witness to psychological health makes it more, rather than less mysterious.

Once, after listening to a part of this patient's trauma-defying story, I let escape a quite unprofessional question: "Are there a lot of people like you?" I was wondering (and still wonder) whether my work as a psychiatrist has given me an unduly pessimistic expectation of the sort of health that can emerge from desperate circumstances.

After an amused pause, she answered "I hope so!" and we both laughed at the mutual realization that indeed, given the circumstances that prevail for most the world's inhabitants—endemic violence, ceaseless objectification and abandonment of human beings—we had all better hope so.

Reinette was conceived in rape and born while her mother, a paranoid schizophrenic, was hospitalized on a psychiatric ward (she was transferred to obstetrics for the occasion). By age five this same mother had tried to kill her by choking her, but less lethal and more confusing treatment was constant during her mother's frequent relapses into profound mental illness. The patient recalls that her mother would apply pancake make-up to make them both appear more "white"; this sort of behavior was a harbinger of more extreme actions such as an attempt to gouge out the little girl's eyes. Social service documents that I reviewed record an instance of mother and daughter being found wandering the city, both unclothed, and note the poignant detail that the child had only one shoe on.

During periods of relative sanity Reinette's mother did her best to love her, but she was alone and unable to protect her daughter from other dangers, among them two much older half brothers. From ages ten to twelve the patient was sexually abused, including intercourse, by one of these brothers, himself also mentally ill. This brother became emotionally dependent on her ("I was the grown-up") and once stabbed himself and crawled into her bed to die. (This attempt failed. He later successfully suicided by jumping out a window.)

Both older brothers tried at different times to rape their mother. Reinette witnessed each of these episodes; they are among the strongest of her memories, always available in vivid detail ("It's there all the time; I just *choose* not to think about it," she replied matter-of-factly to my inquiry). But the State only took action during another of her mother's prolonged psychiatric hospitalizations, when she was thirteen.

Over the next several years in State custody, Reinette was placed in a succession of five different foster homes, three of which proved physically and/or sexually abusive. By that time, though clearly showing intellectual gifts, she had become insolent and rebellious. At eighteen her emancipation was marked by a sanguine discharge note from social services. By nineteen she was bulimic, sexually promiscuous, and addicted to cocaine.

I will not detail the means by which this young woman extricated herself from the predictable fate her story scripts out for her. They were gradual and did not involve the conversion experience, religious or secular, that one might expect in any retelling of the familiar myth of "up from adversity." Reinette was never saved by anything or anyone. She was, in important ways, saved from the beginning by a power which—whatever its source—emerged steadily and consistently from within herself, as I will illustrate piecemeal below. Her decisions after freeing herself from addiction were, in fact, continuous with others she had been making all along: intuitive responses which kept her personhood intact despite all the assaults inflicted on her by others and by herself.

Many of the traditional biographical elements of those who "transcend their origins" are notably absent from her history. Reinette was physically attractive (and "white-looking," in her mother's words) and intelligent, but she did not reside within the shelter of any stably functional family or community for very long. No outside adult stepped credibly into her life in a mentor or surrogate-parent role. She believed in God, but no unambiguous religious faith provided absolute moral guidance. And today her thriving does not seem to require a grandiose perception of herself, nor does she unrealistically idealize or devalue those around her. Reinette is rooted in her painful history but does not advertise it.

The sort of therapy Reinette told me she wanted was help with the present and immediate future: deciding what to do about her mother, of whom she was now legal guardian, when she moved out of state; acculturating to a profession still dominated by white men. She did *not* want to elaborate a victim identity based on her history or to "work on her trauma." She had no need for an idealized parent and specifically wanted no special treatment as a minority woman. "The last time I tried to go to a therapist, they heard my story and wanted to rescue me," she said.

I started out with the usual assumptions. As she told me of the events of the past week, I would look for, and not find, the interpersonal distortions and "defensive operations" generally found in chronically traumatized individuals who enter therapy. Instead, I heard healthy coping, with lots of humor. So I took to comparing what I heard to what I might have expected out loud, by way of encouragement as well as a muted further inquiry.

She also wanted to hear about me and found my reticence about "self-disclosure" a little odd, maybe even offensive. I explained the importance of boundaries and my concern not to establish a pattern, however subtle, of violating hers. "If you ever tried anything I'd kill you," she assured me. So we often ended up telling each other parallel stories, commiserating about the vagaries of interracial friendship, academic or medical politics, and so on. Periodically I would ask if she found these conversations helpful; they felt almost casual, yet sometimes she arrived out of breath rushing to get here on time.

For me, two consistent themes emerged from these "casual" conversations and the occasional glimpses of narrative history into which we would stumble from time to time. I will describe each of these, which I came to see as defining elements of her health, in turn.

The first I might call the refusal of objectification—that is, an insistence on remaining a human subject, a center of autonomous consciousness and power, rather than allowing herself to be made into an object by others. This refusal was most starkly visible in her account of the sexualized, sadistic beatings she regularly received at the hands of her first foster mother, at around age thirteen. Throughout these, Reinette told me, she did her best to maintain eye contact—to look into her abuser's eyes—and not to cry. How could she have known, at that age, the symbolic importance of her act: how "I contact" (a pun I can't resist) would keep her a person, not an acquiescent prop in her foster mother's sick internal script? There is a West African tradition, probably not unique, that one sees through the eyes into the soul of another. Legend has it that captured slaves looked piercingly into the eyes of their captors. All this my patient learned years later.

Overt abuse is one thing, but objectification in the form of "help" is sometimes harder to see. At fourteen, one of Reinette's series of court-appointed social workers decided to invite her home to dinner with the social worker's own family. No doubt moved by this gifted teenager's plight, the worker told Reinette that it would be good for her to "experience a normal family." But Reinette's vision was better than the social worker's; somehow she intuited the destructive precedent that accepting this invitation would have set. She would not make herself an object of pity. "I'm not your urban renewal project," she replied.

One era's vehicle for self-serving charity becomes the next era's candidate for empowerment; liberalism moves in mysterious ways. Patronized as a black girl in the 1980s, Reinette now finds that a female African-American intellectual in the 1990s can be a hot commodity. And she refuses this inverted scale of "value" just as instinctively.

A particularly instructive example of her mental processing came up when she was participating in a panel discussion of a new black filmmaker's work. A fellow panelist, who was white, risked some critical comments and was promptly assailed by minorities in the audience. Reinette thought the panelist's points were well taken, and said so. The gun-barrels of political correctness were now trained upon her. A black woman in the audience invoked moral authority as she spoke: "I come from Alabama, and...."

Though she didn't say it out loud, Reinette inwardly lampooned the level of discourse that was developing. "So, do you have a banjo on your knee?" she said to herself. She then proceeded aloud to defend her fellow panelist.

This last anecdote puts us at two removes from Reinette's refusal to be objectified by the abusive foster mother, but the principle is identical in all three of the above examples. With the social worker, she refused to be objectified in an ostensibly "benign" or "charitable" way, because she saw the surrender of power hidden by the worker's good will: that most important of powers, the ability to define one's own reality. With the fellow panelist, Reinette refused the temptation to racial revenge; refused to "pile on" to the white critic along with her supposed ally, the woman from Alabama. Here, she refused to objectify another, seeing that such a discourse would make herself, the triumphant African-American woman, an object too...just the object that happened to have the power at that moment. The underlying value scale of rightness-by-race would survive unquestioned.

With her inward quip about the banjo, Reinette grasped intuitively a fundamental philosophical tenet that thinkers through the ages keep trying to spell out for us. As Hegel put it in his dialectic of the Master and the Slave, the master is himself enslaved by the structure of slavery. More recently, Jiddu Krishnamurti said it another way: "There is only one relationship. The relationship to others *is* the relationship to the self." If we objectify another on the basis of difference, we also objectify and dehumanize what is different or unknown within ourselves.

The second thematic element of Reinette's remarkable health was a relentless drive to find and use, or make and use, those relationships and experiences which she needed in order to develop. Upon giving up her addiction to cocaine without the help of the twelve steps ("NA meetings were just a good place to score"), Reinette decided to find her mother. This chronically psychotic woman had drifted to another state where she was under public guardianship. Rather naively, Reinette moved in with her, hoping to "work out" what had happened in the family and obtain validation from the mother who had been unable to protect her. I was reminded of Harlow's famous experiments of the 1960s. Chimpanzee mothers who were themselves raised in isolation were found to ignore or brutalize their children. But the offspring kept trying: "One of the most interesting findings was that despite the consistent punishment, the babies persisted in their attempts to make maternal contact."

Even with better psychiatric care orchestrated by her daughter, who obtained guardianship, it became painfully clear that the older, schizophrenic woman would never be restored to the level of emotional functioning necessary for the kind of resolution Reinette wanted. But Reinette found things to love and admire about her mother and felt loved by her, even if not truly known. Seeing her mother's limitations for what they were and grieving them made her own childhood more comprehensible and did have healing value.

To choose certain life experiences is, of course, not to choose others. One such instructive, and negative, decision occurred at a point in her education when Reinette was considering a career in the social services. Classic "rescue fantasies," wherein she, empowered by professional authority, would go in and right the kinds of wrongs she had herself experienced, were operating to motivate her. As a part of her course work, she was assigned to an internship at a battered women's shelter.

I have known and worked with other trauma survivors whose response to the overwhelming and re-traumatizing experience of such front-lines social service work has been in fact to enter the mental health field or related areas. Consciously or unconsciously they are drawn toward the attempt to master their own emotional turmoil through identifying with and trying to help their clients. Sometimes—particularly with competent supervision and personal psychotherapy—this moth-to-the-flame approach can work. Without a careful cultivation of self-awareness, though, this choice becomes "reaction formation," potentially dangerous to clients and professionals alike.

Reinette's response was different, and she recounted it with characteristic simplicity. "I was just hearing my own story again and again," she told me. "I thought, *I don't need to hear this again and again!*"

So in the rest of her schooling she focused on different areas which fascinated her intellectually, feeling that her altruism would best be expressed in other, safer contexts. In the present, I noticed that Reinette preferred to remain vulnerable and not to steel herself against anything; she let herself be affected by her friends' everyday problems, by her husband's illness at one point, by her own migraines. This vulnerability was incompatible with any kind of reactive mastery of her life, yet somehow she succeeded and thrived.

Such "trauma work" as we ended up doing was occasional and unsystematic, yet we both knew something was happening. I later got an unusual confirmation of this from the osteopathic physician who had originally referred her to me. Apparently, a chronic muscle spasm which had been unresponsive to manipulative therapy cleared up spontaneously during our year of psychotherapy. It had been related, the osteopath thought, to yet another episode of physical abuse whose story I had never heard.

The stories I did eventually hear in some detail—after the typical beginning of small talk—were those of each brother's sexual assault on Reinette's mother. I still recall her description of her and her mother sitting beside each other, both trembling before the terrifying madness of one of these young men; how Reinette so wanted to protect her mother and have mother protect her, and how abjectly helpless she was to obtain safety for either of them. After relating this episode simply, neither detached from nor drowning in affect, she looked intensely and directly at me. "What makes a person do something like that?" she asked. She was a sophisticated person who knew, cognitively, that there could be no one simple answer to the question. I admired the fact that she would let herself ask it from the depth of her feeling.

In a few seconds I reviewed, and rejected, various possible explanations I might have offered. One attempt might focus on the disease Schizophrenia, its delusional distortions, its disinhibition or misdirection of affect and instinct. Another might speculate on the origins of her brother's rage against his mother. Neither these, nor others—indeed, not even the idea of offering an explanation—felt right. So I looked back at Reinette and said, "I don't know." And then, as I had so often done in lieu of explanation or technique, I found myself telling a parallel story of my own.

I must have been seven. Dad had found my seventeen-year-old brother "parking" with his girlfriend (they are now thirty years married) and tried to stop them, but my brother drove off. When he returned to the house later, a fistfight started between these two physically powerful men. This was no ordinary occurrence in our family; I was terrified looking on, and my loyalties quite naturally lay with my father, who was at first getting the worst of it. I ran to my dresser drawer and got out my hunting knife with which to stab my brother if need be. But I stood there shaking instead until my father finally rallied and won without me. (They are now the best of friends, and I still carry this memory.)

As I told my story, I could see that Reinette was moved by the little boy's predicament; any "quantitative" comparison I might make between this isolated incident and the years of abuse and violence she had experienced didn't seem to matter to her. She was with me, emotionally, as I told this story, which somehow seemed the most appropriate response I could make to hearing her own.

It turned out that I had a point to make about my own experience of being with her. "I've been trained to spin out theories and explanations," I said to her in conclusion. "But trying to explain what your brother did would be like getting out my little knife when I was a boy." In other words, both of us as children, and even now as adults, were finally helpless. Our knives and our theories and our defenses were no match for the raw forces of love/hate raging uncontrolled around us. Both of us saw the truth of this. Sitting together in my office, in that helpless place, acknowledging and naming it for what it was, and not applying techniques or theories against the terror and the mystery—this alone seemed the best way for me to respect the life force contained in this remarkable woman.

CASE 7:
THE NEW COVENANT

This was a young man's case. I even kept count of the sessions! As one grows older in psychotherapy, energy, idealism and the impulse to "make something happen" are tempered by other principles. If I had not been full of the spirit of adventure when I encountered this man, I would have missed the almost poetic softening of his character, as well as a synchronistic surprise at the end.

This is the only case I saved from an early phase of absorption with Milton Erickson's unorthodox methods and an attempt to achieve "prowess" in using them. It was first presented at the Fourth Annual San Diego Conference on Hypnotic and Strategic Interventions (1988), during the heyday of the Ericksonian movement. Its tone is admittedly a bit didactic and self-congratulatory. I include it, though, because the contact the two of us made in this therapy was truly surprising and my part of it did not feel manipulative or procedural in nature (as most of my work of that time, in retrospect, did).

"The New Covenant: Elements of Personal Contact in a Challenging Case of Depression" was finally published, minus most of the Ericksonian verbiage, in the May 1994 *Psychiatric Times.*

As opportunities for engaging in intensive, individualized psychotherapy continue to decline in favor of standardized short-term approaches, those of us who have given substantial parts of our careers to the former work feel a need to assert and to preserve what we have learned. In this spirit I offer the following case.

The standard treatments sometimes fail. When this happens, a creative collaboration which enlists the unique interests and aptitudes of both therapist and patient is called for. Because such work *by definition* eludes replicability and quantification, its effectiveness has been ascribed to "non-specific factors." Appreciation of or empathy with the patient become anecdotal and unfathomable abstractions. But if therapists truly appreciate or empathize with their patients, they do so in specific ways for specific reasons.

Milton Erickson invited therapists to intervene in a context created by the patient's problem rather than that of a preconceived theory or technique:

> "Since whatever patients bring into the office is in some way both a part of them and a part of their problem, the patient should be viewed with a sympathetic eye appraising the totality which confronts the therapist ... Sometimes— in fact, many more times than is realized —therapy can be firmly established only by the utilization of silly, absurd, irrational, and contradictory manifestations. One's professional dignity is not involved, but one's professional competence is." [*Innovative Hypnotherapy*, p. 213]

Jung put it more succinctly: "We need a different language for each patient."

In presenting the following case, I will not try to prove that creativity was the only factor in our success. Skeptics (including myself) will be able to construct alternative explanations, some of a more biological nature. But, at a minimum, the psychotherapeutic innovations here described strengthened an alliance that was able to hold the patient in treatment long enough for biological improvement to occur.

When Errol, sixty, first arrived in my office, the only cheerful thing I could discern about him was his jaunty, closely trimmed moustache, reminiscent of the movie heroes of a bygone era. It would have to sustain me for many weeks. His ashen, drawn face and slouched posture corresponded to the monotone of his factual, affectless answers. He had been depressed for three years, since losing his life savings in a business operation. At an age when he had expected to retire comfortably, he had been forced to hire himself out to do hard physical labor using tradesman's skills he had learned earlier in life. He needed to support not only himself, but a small child and a younger, second wife.

Errol described the onset of his depression, after the financial catastrophe, as "feeling like a five-year-old boy in a 200 pound body." He recalled crying uncontrollably, feeling physically sick and exhausted. After a few weeks of this, he consulted his internist, who did the usual "rule-out" workup and then placed Errol on high doses of a tricyclic antidepressant. This enabled him to function, but left him sexually impotent, forgetful and chronically drowsy. He would drag himself to work, endure it, go home and collapse on a chair until falling asleep. One attempt at stopping the tricyclic on his own resulted in a full relapse. The internist, who saw Errol briefly every six months, refilled the prescription and never referred him to a psychiatrist, despite the chronicity of his depression.

Errol finally sought therapy on the authority of a magazine article he had seen which, fortunately, mentioned something about psychotherapy being of use in the treatment of depression. Authority, as I would find, was something Errol had a lifelong pattern of trusting rather too completely—the authority of his internist (backed by the institution of medicine) and of the magazine (the institution of academic clinical psychology) were only two recent examples. During a twenty-five-year career in an elite branch of the military, his life had involved both following and enforcing rules and regulations which were assumed to be trustworthy. What bothered him most about losing his money was not the large sum involved but having been cleverly tricked out of it in a way which fully conformed with certain regulations Errol had agreed to. He obsessed a great deal about having thus been cheated "fairly," and was frustrated by the slow pace and high cost of his efforts to pursue the matter legally. (At this juncture in the history-taking, anger fleetingly enlivened the man.)

More information came from Errol's wife's therapist, who had referred Errol to me. His wife described him as cold, punitive, frequently yelling, spending no time with her or the child. Any energy or spare time was taken up with his intense involvement in a fundamentalist religious sect. This involvement, which he had not mentioned to me himself, revealed the ultimate authority in Errol's life—the literal authority of the Bible. The religious interest had intensified since the onset of his illness. His wife's opinion was that religion, rather than the antidepressant, "kept him going." Her therapy often focused on her problems with him, but he had refused an invitation to enter conjoint work.

I looked for developmental explanations for Errol's attitude but drew a blank. Childhood and family were described in distant, simplistically positive terms. The parents had been "loving," the family "stable" and conflict-free. I was never to learn more of it than this. Errol entered the service at eighteen and stayed through three wars, including some combat experience which he did not feel affected him adversely. He had a "poor" first marriage, which lasted thirty years, and from which he had grown children. He was finally divorced following a long separation. He later retired from the military, entered business, and married again not long before the depression occurred. There had been no psychiatric contact. Medical authority had, however, saved his life about a year before his financial misfortune. A potentially fatal cancer was found in a routine radiologic study before it had spread, and it was surgically cured.

This man was going to be hard to work with. I suspected that his willingness to trust the impersonal authority of institutions, the Bible, or accepted medical/psychological procedures compensated for an inability to trust individuals.

Five years into my psychotherapeutic career I was little more than a novice, but I am not sure that was a bad thing. The weariness of experience and a fuller practice might have led me to give up before any rapport-building ability I may have acquired took hold. As it was, it took me the first ten of our thirty-seven sessions just to arrive at a way of working with this man.

While I floundered, Errol sat like a rock, volunteering nothing, showing no emotion. He was unable or unwilling to respond to the usual inquiries, and there were no dreams.

Hoping to establish myself as a reliable helper in at least one sphere, I focused on medication side effects. Fortunately, a sizeable reduction in the dose restored Errol's ability to ejaculate, and his memory, without an increase in depressive symptoms. The wisdom of accepted psychiatric practice was thus confirmed. But Errol remained uninterested in sex (which, he told me, was not like him) and more generally, in life, and we reached a bottom limit below which he couldn't go without relapsing into his original full-blown depression.

Sessions continued to stagnate. I abandoned psychodynamics in favor of a variety of recently-learned hypnotic techniques which I will not detail here. The hypnotic work was not particularly fruitful. Errol couldn't collaborate with me for very long; he wouldn't risk exploring his own spontaneous imagery or sensory experience but instead wanted to have me direct him explicitly. "You're the professional," he would say. That kept me in my safe, impersonally authoritative place. The idea of "healing from within," such a commonplace even then, was utterly alien to him, and if invoked just added to the evidence of my own incompetence.

Finally we recovered a dream fragment which revealed another, unconscious aspect of his reaction to me. Errol was in an office meeting with a young, inexperienced accountant who seemed overwhelmed by Errol's financial situation and was considering referring his case elsewhere! This unconscious perception about my feelings was of course accurate. But the dream also showed that beneath his seeming defiance, real hope that I could help him was giving way to the fear of abandonment. For fear of making matters worse, I did not broach this interpretation then. I would get another chance.

Errol asked me to meet with his wife after the first ten sessions. She described his religious involvement, which she felt oppressed her and their child. This particular creed, as Errol observed it, emphasized a future paradise. One got there by avoiding undue concern with the affections and material pleasures of this life. Hours upon hours of Bible study would make it possible to precisely anticipate events leading to the end of the world. If the wife persisted in her lack of involvement, she would not join her husband in paradise. Whenever Errol felt well enough to attend, he brought his young daughter along to lengthy religious meetings in hopes that she, at least, might be saved.

Errol had not yet discussed his religious life with me, but he *had* asked that I speak to his wife about him in order to "shed some light on the situation." Now I had an opening, and I asked him to explain his beliefs. He began to expound upon "biblical" doctrine in an angry, animated way, bitterly criticizing our secularized culture with its worldly attractions. He did not believe, for example, in the giving of gifts from one person to another. To honor someone, he believed, one should only give to the church in that person's name. Otherwise the misguided giver and recipient would both be sinning by placing their friendship above love for God.

I drew Errol's attention to a Christmas card in the office sent to me by a former patient. "Do you mean to say God is dishonored by my accepting a card from this fine person?" I asked. "Exactly," he said. Picking the gift up, I asked if, according to biblical teaching, I had therefore best destroy the card. Errol looked alarmed and started to qualify himself, saying that he couldn't speak for my situation. "But isn't biblical doctrine *true* independent of any particular situation?" I insisted. Of course, Errol had to agree. I tore up the card and ended the session abruptly. My action had been entirely spontaneous; all I knew was that I had, myself, felt angry.

In the following (twelfth) session, I told Errol, truthfully, that I was interested in the Bible, but I regretted what I had done with the gift. In retrospect, following through on Errol's literal "rule of law" had shown me directly how destructive authority, the letter of the law had become to him (through the business reversal) and now to those around him (through religious dogma). My anger was not at him but at (paraphrasing II Corinthians 3:6) "the letter that killeth," as opposed to "the spirit that giveth life."

I suggested that we spend some time studying the Bible together as a way for me to better understand his point of view. In his blunted way Errol was excited by this proposal. Perhaps he saw a possibility of converting me to his beliefs.

If Errol had established any glimmer of risky, personal trust in me, it could now be safely subordinated to a truly reliable Higher Authority. We agreed to take turns assigning passages from the Bible to discuss in therapy. This was to be our "technique" for the following twelve sessions.

Errol used these biblical sessions to set forth the key tenets of his own way of believing. For him the Bible was a code book predicting future events and secondarily an infallible guide to behavior. He showed no literary or metaphorical appreciation of it. "Why would God produce a scripture which needs deciphering; which makes prediction so difficult?" I often asked. "I don't question God's motivations," he would say.

I chose passages whose sense seemed to contradict each other. I would contrast, for example, the exuberant sexuality of the *Song of Solomon* with Pauline writings espousing celibacy, or the loving Jesus of the Gospels with the murderous vision of the Son of Man in *Revelation*. Though Errol was wily in eluding "literal" contradictions, he had to admit that the tone in these passages was very different. Why would God include them all in His book? "I don't question God's motivations."

Errol's active involvement in this phase of the therapy implied an overall improvement in his depression; this was confirmed by a phone call from his wife. He seemed more alive, more emotionally available to the family, and more flexible in small ways. In session, our verbal sparring revealed Errol's quick wit and an inquiring mind which underlay his refusal to question. I wanted to protect the improvement and so was careful not to mention it.

For me the culmination of our biblical work came in session twenty-three. The night before I had selected a passage from *Exodus* (32:7-14; quotes are King James' version) which I knew from Freud's classic essay on authority, "The Moses of Michaelangelo." In this scene, God and Moses confer atop Mount Sinai after the delivery of the Ten Commandments. God learns that the Israelites below have begun to worship a golden calf and decides to destroy them. "Now therefore let me alone, that my wrath may wax hot against them, and that I may consume them" (32:10). Moses intercedes with God, reminding him of the mighty works whereby he delivered them from Egypt and of his promises to Abraham and Isaac. "And the Lord repented of the evil which he thought to do unto his people" (32:14).

"Here in the Bible itself is a man who questioned God's motivations," I pointed out to Errol. As a literal believer, he had no choice but to admit this, and he left the session appearing confused. God's contemplated action would have paralleled my destruction of the Christmas card in session eleven, but Moses' questioning prevented this. God Himself proved capable of repentance *before* rather than (as in my case) after the fact. In developmental language, this constitutes good-enough parental empathy. The implicit suggestion for Errol: "You can meet your needs better by questioning, rather than passively accepting, authority. As an adult, you have this choice."

In the following (twenty-fourth) session, Errol reported a dream of meeting a young man with an Italian name who was lost in a large city, asking *him* for directions. This obvious reference to me was an elaboration of the earlier accountant figure. This time, building on Exodus, I aimed to interpret it. I asked Errol in what way I seemed to him to be lost. He replied that after our last session he'd wondered what I was doing with his therapy; he doubted that my training had included a course in using the Bible. I applauded this questioning, which clearly evidenced the development of a stronger internal locus of control. "Now that you've seen Moses question God's authority, you can question mine," I observed. I then reviewed his life-long pattern of accepting authority, from military to religion to internist to me. He laughed as he recognized this.

In the succeeding nine sessions (twenty-five through thirty-four), Errol indeed did take more control of his therapy. He opened up the details of his present life to me (often with the aid of prepared lists) and asked me for comments and suggestions. Emphasizing my own fallibility, I made some, and we collaborated in approaching the practical problems he faced. I frequently made reference to biblical precepts—the "common language" we had developed—and phrased suggestions in Christian terms. The use of the Bible respected Errol's conception of divine authority while allowing him to progressively experience the strengthening of his own autonomy on a practical, everyday level. I hoped to shift Errol's religious focus more to the present but had no interest in undermining his specific beliefs about the future. Thus, he could treat his wife and child kindly *now* (following Jesus' example) rather than seek only to get them into the future paradise.

This phase of our work was more counseling than psychotherapy. I felt like a well-meaning friend, not a new authority figure. Errol seemed to be unlearning "learned helplessness." By session thirty-four, his residual depression was almost entirely gone. Family and sexual relationships were vigorous and satisfying, if not conflict-free. Errol continued to try and recover his financial losses through legal means, but he was no longer obsessed about having been cheated, nor was he waiting for a legal victory—some final vindication in the realm of impersonal, judicial authority of which there was no assurance—to restore his self-esteem. We had further tapered the tricyclic below a standard therapeutic range, but a persistent sleep disturbance made it necessary to continue the medication (for three more years, it would turn out).

A skeptic might say that lowering this medication dose was my major therapeutic intervention. Whatever the cause for Errol's improvement, both of us felt that regular weekly therapy was no longer needed.

The Bible once again proved a natural way of approaching a session: this time, our final session. My choice of passages was intuitive, rather than engineered, and was made the night before based on my modest knowledge of scripture and my feelings about Errol. Looking back I would say that he was emerging from an Old Testament world of authority into the New Covenant of Christian charity (i.e., interpersonal reciprocity); perhaps I wanted him in some way to internalize his route. All of the passages were from the Old Testament.

I began with snippets from *Proverbs*, that compendium of timeless Jewish wisdom. I aimed to ratify some of Errol's practical discoveries in the latter part of our therapy when we had worked in counseling mode. Examples: "A false balance is abomination to the Lord: but a just weight is his delight" [11:1]. "The liberal soul shall be made fat: and he that watereth shall be watered also himself" [11:25].

To conclude, I went to *Judges* 14, the beginning of the story of Samson. On his way to take a Philistine wife, the young Samson tears a lion apart with his bare hands. Returning to the carcass later, he finds a bees' nest within it and eats the honey inside. Later he challenges his companions to decipher a riddle. "And he said unto them, Out of the eater came forth meat, and out of the strong came forth sweetness" (14:14).

I emphasize again that I chose this passage spontaneously and intuitively. Today I read its message as follows: Interpersonally, as an autonomous adult, Errol could question authority (kill the lion) and obtain nurturance (eat the honey). Intrapsychically, he could allow himself to be sweet (forgiving, flexible) as well as strong.

As we finished, Errol reported with some astonishment that he had studied the same passage in *Judges* the previous night and was to be responsible for expounding upon the same chapters of *Proverbs* from which I had read the following week!

Such examples of "synchronicity" as a byproduct of therapeutic rapport are impossible to study systematically but are as old as psychotherapy itself. Rather than dwell upon any mystical dimension to this highly improbable event, I simply noted that such occurrences had been observed before in similar situations. I advised Errol that these passages may indeed have some special significance for him. My afterthought as I write is: for me as well. And so we ended the work.

In a follow-up medication visit two months later Errol told me, "My whole outlook has changed." He was free of all his original symptoms. He remained active in his church and somewhat rigid in style, but he found life and particularly his marriage very satisfying. His sense of humor was particularly enjoyable. These gains were maintained in further visits one, two, and three years later.

Biased as I am toward mistrusting the forces that are fast standardizing our field, I found, in the American Psychiatric Association's *Practice Guideline for the Treatment of Major Depression* (1993), unlikely support for my work with Errol:

> "In practice, psychiatrists use a combination or synthesis of various approaches and strategies; these in turn are determined by and individually tailored to each patient on the basis of that person's particular conditions and coping capacities. Furthermore, in actual application the techniques and the therapist-patient relationship are powerfully intertwined."

There are many ways to conceptualize my work with Errol. Winnicott might say that the Bible became a transitional space within which he could renegotiate the relationship of self and object. Aaron Beck might point to the frequent challenging of negative "cognitive schemata" in the therapy. Freud himself might remark that the Old Testament God of *Exodus* provided a nicely oedipal authority who did the right thing at the right time.

Conceptualizations are after the fact; they abstract from selected aspects of a far more complex (or is it more simple?) reality that exists in the consulting room. The point is that neither these authorities, nor any treatment manual, nor the recent APA guidelines, actually generated my interventions with Errol. Instead they emerged from a mysterious intersubjectivity; from the spontaneous willingness to take a patient in his own terms and his willingness to take me in mine.

PART II:
SUPERVISION AND
SELF-DISCLOSURE

INTRODUCTION TO PART II

I love to hear myself talk. This becomes a problem in my line of work, where listening is so essential. My efforts to contain myself as a therapist have been successful enough to earn the ultimate accolade from some patients—"You're too quiet!"—but I do let loose upon supervisees when I get the chance, warning them to interrupt me as needed.

All of the essays in Part II evolved from supervisory dialogues (and monologues). I converted these particular ones to written form because 1) I especially liked them and found myself repeating parts of them, and 2) supervisees or others (i.e. someone, somewhere) found them interesting and/or helpful.

Without exception, all of my trainees have been sincere in their desire to connect with their patients and to help them and know them. And to varying degrees all have sometimes been overwhelmed by the amount and depth of illness and emotional pain in the world. They learn there is no bottom to it.

Since many of my supervisees have been psychiatric residents or newly trained clinicians from other disciplines, their prior exposure to the classical literature of psychotherapy has been minimal. The analytic language in which much of it is written is as remote to them as Elizabethan English. Thus, one constant aim of my teaching has been to pass on as much as I can of the remarkable insights of some of the Old Masters—Jung, Balint, Winnicott, Horney, Semrad—so these young clinicians will not have to reinvent the wheel when their training in today's standardized cognitive-behavioral techniques fails them.

I wage an ongoing guerilla war against these new orthodoxies while trying simultaneously to remain open to the value and real innovation contained in some of them. (Marcia Linehan's "Dialectical Behavior Therapy" and the new cognitive neuropsychology are two examples.) And I try to model integrative thinking about the revolutionary new psychoactive medications and how they influence (not bypass) patients' individual psychologies. This integrative effort has been absolutely necessary to maintain credibility in this past "decade of the brain" with therapists and patients who

51

have grown up in the psychopharmacological era. But I have stopped short of any premature "synthesis," choosing to synthesize only in miniature, about individual patients.

Most important, I have stressed these beginning therapists' need to learn what kind of therapist *they* can be. Each needs to find out what kinds of interventions fit his or her own personality, rather than succumb to the procedural mentality—the "see one, do one, teach one" of medical school—which turns therapists and their patients into collections of interchangeable parts.

My supervisees did not all get the same supervisor. Like anyone who has been in the business long enough, I have gone through cycles of idealism and disillusionment regarding psychotherapy, and these cycles are variously reflected in the essays in Part II. (The best I have managed toward an explanation of them is the piece called "Raffaela's Hug.") Inherent in the therapeutic enterprise is a polarity of orientations which I have called Romantic vs. Tragic. It might equally be called, with only slight exaggeration, Manic vs. Depressive.

Someone who ought to know (William James? Alfred North Whitehead?) once wrote that "A great Truth is one whose opposite is also a great Truth." Romantic optimism is a perennially dominant theme in the culture and literature of psychotherapy. In a jaundiced mood I call it the Star Wars approach: "Trust your feelings, Luke!" Just remove the downed branches from the stream of life and flow will be restored; the patient's life force will heal her from within. "I once was lost but now I'm found," as we regularly sing at our American Academy of Psychotherapists meetings.

The opposite Truth informs the Tragic or pessimistic view of our work: "I once was found but now I'm lost." Such a view tends to emphasize much more the enormous fact of innate temperament and the need to adapt as best as we can to what cannot be changed or re-parented out of existence. In the Tragic perspective, affect cannot always be trusted—it can potentially kill us as well as heal us—and that Romantic whipping boy, cognition, sometimes offers the only salvation (though that is a Romantic term; salvation in this view is only relative). Here, verbal thought can be a freeing thing, not just a defense or a block.

One learns to honor and respect patients' defenses as one's career goes on. The Romantic view, lovely as it is, conceals a basic non-acceptance of the Other. It is always wanting to heal away defenses and remake the Other in its own Romantic image. The Tragic view offers the possibility of enjoying and appreciating the Other *as Other*. Yet the ability of the Romantic approach to sometimes cure is undeniable. Left unconscious, these two opposite therapeutic Truths find natural homes in different stages of one therapist's career, or in therapists of different temperaments. The few master practitioners I have known are sometimes able to hold the Whole Truth within their healing and helping work, keeping both opposite principles simultaneously in conscious view. I have never fully succeeded in this, but teaching and writing about it has helped me try.

THE THAW

We like to think that there are rules to follow that will both keep us safe and help us to heal our patients. We talk about "keeping our boundaries" and with good reason. But the reality of therapeutic boundaries is that few patients get better until these boundaries are crossed in some way or another. The teaching of rigid rules prevents us from talking honestly about the inevitable risk involved in initiating or accepting boundary crossings and how to take that risk in a responsible way.

The editors at *Psychiatric Times* liked this piece enough to put it right up front in the February 1999 issue, a rare treat for me.

Many of us enter medicine because we want to take care of people and be thanked, even loved, for it. This motivation sustains us in our efforts to heal. How much should we allow it to bring us closer to the patient at hand, and how wary need we be that such closeness may impede our ability to help him or her in a professional way? Supervision in psychodynamic psychotherapy gives our trainees the chance to develop the critical discernment they will need to make this judgment, patient after patient, through the rest of their clinical careers.

The patient has brought my resident supervisee a gift. I have painted such things myself, taking up my watercolors in January or February as much in prayer as in description. Black water is showing here and there through the ice; on the stream banks, packets of snow darken toward the green or brown underneath. This is an emotional state, an earliest of hopes, known to all who make their home in wintery latitudes. And in this patient's life the relationship with his therapist has triggered the thaw.

I have already learned this supervisee possesses a natural empathic attunement. He is a Kohutian by temperament without having yet read Kohut. When the painting his patient had brought in, ostensibly to "share," was left behind—a surprise at session's end, inscribed as a gift—the supervisee (who genuinely liked it) hung it up. And he did not insist on belaboring the attempt at interpretation next session. Instead, he allowed the patient to noncommittally deflect the gentle question, "Does this painting have anything to do with how you feel?" This beginning therapist intuits a healing value in accepting, for now, the positive transference in which he is cast, not inaccurately, as a benignly approving figure. But he also knows that he has made a decision and wants to weigh its implications with me.

This resident has no need for the illusion that there is a "right" thing to do here. In this he differs from many of his peers, including myself at his stage of training. How well I can remember the secret feeling of relief when my own supervisor would reassert such an illusion, even when he told me, "What you did was a major error." At least there was safety in some way: his way.

I have since learned on my own that, nine times out of ten, there is no "right" thing to do, and even to be thankful for that fact. Therapy is a series of more or less controlled mistakes, and if there are no mistakes there can be no therapy—only a sterile procedure in which patients learn to successively approximate an unerring authority figure and are thus sealed into implicit inferiority. This may help them adapt, but please, let's call it something else.

When I read Winnicott, I learned that this point of view is Winnicottian. Its central question to the therapist is, "Which kind of hole would you rather dig yourself out of?" When we look at all of our interventions as mistakes (i.e., the natural results of being a human Other in our patients' lives), then the operating-room anxiety evaporates. Therapy becomes a series of branch points ("bifurcating universes," in the Californian phrase), and a different anxiety follows upon the knowledge that uncertainty can never be banished, the last artery never tied off.

What sort of hole is this resident's natural inclination digging for him? He does not know this patient all that well as yet; their relationship remains untested. What risk is there in not insisting on a thorough, conscious look at the gift and its interpersonal meaning in the therapy?

By finding the patient's painting worthy to hang in his office, my supervisee has added something of his real-world self to the positive transference. He has registered his own judgment about the picture's quality, providing an external source of self-esteem for the patient. Will more insistent demands upon the therapist's positive regard follow on this first, tentative gesture? And what happens when the resident cannot wholeheartedly congratulate or approve of some future action of the patient's? Should he "fake it" and skirt the issue "for the patient's good" developmentally? (Borderline spectrum patients tend to see right through such paternalism, yet may paradoxically feel that the therapist, having accepted the gift, "owes" it to them.)

At what point will the resident risk interrupting the "safe place," the holding environment this relationship has created? When will he judge himself and the patient ready to enter the other side—the depriving, humiliating side—of the transference that is building? By then will the patient be able to tolerate the Fall from Eden, the threat to what has probably been (from what we know of the history) the best and most validating relationship he has ever experienced? Or will this particular patient try to reinstate/refute Perfect Care with ever more extreme regression: ER visits, suicide gestures, medication "refractoriness," or noncompliance?

By this time I have given my poor supervisee quite a scare.

But any unitary hazard can become too comfortable; the resident may get the impression that the "right way" to go is as simple as girding his loins, insisting on insight, being ready to confront unrealistic dependency and set limits when necessary. So I switch to what the risks of a more questioning response to the gift might be. Would raising the possibility of "owing" something—any hint that there could be the slightest manipulativeness in the hopeful act of gift giving—drive the patient away literally, or perhaps deeper into his illness? Would the resident's application of critical thinking, a refusal to wordlessly accept the painting (and the idealizing projection) further starve the patient's hunger for a mirror: a person capable of sharing the subjective experience of the thaw? (Analysts will have to forgive my mixing of Kohut's metaphors here.)

More simply, would a premature exposure to consciousness blight tender seedlings of optimism about the therapy that are best left under the dirt (as the legendary hypnotherapist Milton Erickson might have warned)?

At this point in my evocation of the possibilities I digress to explain to the resident the unfashionable concepts of developmental arrest and corrective emotional experience. I tell a story from when I was eight and growing up on Lake Winnepesaukee. Once while my father bought groceries at the local marina I stayed on the dock with the boat and informed a couple of local teenagers that it was (as I believed) "the fastest boat on the lake." They, of course, knew better, but I held to my truth through their heckling until my father returned. "Isn't this the fastest boat on the lake?" I demanded in this now-public forum. He took in the scene, nodded yes to the teenagers solemnly, and as we left the dock he suddenly gunned our outboard motor so that we left in a white wake of speed and glory.

My father had seen that I needed our boat to be the fastest boat (and he the strongest man) on Lake Winnepesaukee that day. I forever thank him for accepting that role, which allowed me to feel proud and safe as I grew.

My supervisee's patient, carrying a history of abandonment and abuse, had never had such a parent. Potentially, the resident's appreciation of his gift might be the first in a series of such "corrective" experiences. The trick would be to avoid the grandiose notion of "re-parenting" and recognize that any such series, at best, is a small nudge to help get development rolling again, like clearing ice from a thawing stream whose real source is elsewhere. Downstream the therapist will hope to manage a gradual-enough disappointment of his patient, so the patient can take power into himself.

Interpretations of the transference at that future point might serve to show how idealizing another disempowers the self. But first one has to experience one's father's boat being fastest, which premature interpretation of the gift could jeopardize.

For therapists in the resident's situation, the most important thing to estimate is whether or not the patient's relational capacity is broken beyond repair. Chronically traumatized patients think in black and white. Some can slowly learn shades of gray wherein the therapist becomes neither demon nor savior but a fallible, if well-meaning, human being. Others will forever swing between polarized alternatives like redemption, abandonment, enslavement, or end with their needles pinned on one such extreme of the emotional meter-gage. I tell trainees who find themselves idealized that their patients can only imagine a good caregiver as the opposite of the abusive or nonexistent caregivers experienced during development. In that sense the patients' imagination is stuck in a place where they themselves have no power and depend abjectly on the Other to create a reality (albeit a less painful reality) for them. Ten or fifty years hence, neuroscience may confirm my conjecture that this black-and-white affective response results from neuronal damage and loss of dense connectivity within the hippocampus—connectivity which normally helps us perceive degrees of relative safety. Thus, functional neuroanatomy might someday describe successful psychotherapy with chronically traumatized individuals as the restoration of adequate interneural connectivity in certain brain areas so that we can again see shades of gray in the relational world.

The arrival of that future golden era seems about as likely as the return of Eden itself, given the current and future limitations of health care resources in the real clinical world. But even if the resident were working in such an ideal climate, I doubt he would be able to tell in any foolproof way whether a given patient is going to be able to use a regression therapeutically or drown himself and his therapist in it. Today we have various "criteria": Has the patient ever had a stable long-term relationship? Is there a family history of major psychiatric illness? and so forth. But after seventeen years of trying to always get this right, I am convinced that using any such set of criteria (or using the functional hippocampal neuroimaging of A.D. 2050) is still going to exclude some people who can benefit from a corrective experience of dependency and include some people who will deteriorate when such an experience is offered.

For life to flow, the crystalline structure of frozen ice must give way. Here lies the risk. The therapist will do his best to manage the rate of the melting, but once a thaw is underway there is always the chance of meltdown: affective flood. Finally, therapist and patient are on their own.

Because his patient's gift opens up such rich questions, I urged my supervisee to ask as many of the faculty as he could for their own opinions on this case. My prediction was that, according to the variety of human temperament, there would be as many opinions as supervisors, all of them worth considering. Certainly in my training this would have been the case.

To my surprise, he reported a unanimous consensus. Accept the gift—don't be a robot in response to this human gesture—but make sure you do talk together a little about what it means. My first reaction was that this represents progress in the field; that we have learned, as a group, to try and avoid the hazards of either extreme position.

But even the prudent outlook of good general psychiatry, if taken too literally, could adversely affect the "learning trajectory" of a resident who seems headed for further destinations in psychodynamic psychotherapy. Will Odysseus hear himself being told to sail straight home, watch out for monsters, and don't talk to any nymphs? So, while he is still closely supervised, I will encourage him (within responsible limits) to follow his natural, empathic impulse and learn how to sail back from there. He then will have a better idea both of that part of the sea and of how to manage his own particular aptitudes and vulnerabilities as a maturing psychotherapist.

HERE ARE THE SCALES

The Spring 1997 issue of *Voices* was devoted to stories and story-telling in psychotherapy; this was my entry. It has been one of my readers' (and my patients') favorites despite its uncompromising message. Perhaps it is easier for people to take because I am talking about my own experience.

I only ever took two formal, paid guitar lessons in my life. But I have recounted them to many patients ever since, because the learning therein transcended the context.

I was feeling ambitious in my early thirties, able to move mountains. Why stop at the rudimentary folk and swing styles with which I amused myself? I wanted to play jazz. So I called a local guitarist whose style I admired and asked if he gave lessons.

Reluctant teachers are generally the most trustworthy. Carlos was in the process of getting out of the music business and into something else. My enthusiasm seemed to make him just slightly wistful. He listened to me play, then we played together. He said a few complimentary things about my phrasing, but my distance from his own free lyricism was all too apparent. He showed me what I would have to do. Here are the Berklee guitar books. Work your way through these. Here are all the scales. Practice them. Here are some interval exercises. Practice them and incorporate them into your solos. Oh and by the way, you're going to have to stop gripping the neck with your thumb. Move it around to the back and don't press so hard. It's the only way you'll have real freedom on the fretboard. Yes, Hendrix played your way, a lot of people play that way—I used to play that way—but now you want to play jazz. Try it this way.

So I tried it in this new position and couldn't play anything; couldn't hold the notes clearly. Everything felt wrong. Carlos shared his experience. When he'd made the switch, all the guys in the band said, "What happened to you?" It took six months to get abreast of where he'd been *before* the different left hand. He was practicing up to five hours a day at the time, working through those Berklee books.

I knew Carlos a little socially, and as I say, he was getting out of the business. He had no motivation to string me along with bite-sized lessons and keep me coming back to pay his fee. These lessons were a favor to me. I know that, be it psychotherapy or music teaching, there are times when it's best not to overwhelm the patient/student and instead to preserve an optimistic tone. Some learners rise to the occasion and take heart when approached in a more incremental way. But if therapists could always do the "initial assessment" as presciently as Carlos did, we would save a lot of time on people like me. This is what you have to do, if you're serious, he reiterated, and you're going to get worse before you get better.

By the end of my second lesson it was clear I wasn't serious about learning to play the jazz guitar. With Carlos' help, it was a conscious choice. I still play a fair amount, by ear, mostly as an excuse to sing. But as for solos, it's rare that I'll even venture a blues scale. I leave that to the serious players or those blessed with a surfeit of raw talent; I stay with what I can do. My thumb remains where it always was.

I reserve this rather harsh story for people who have started to change and are past a point of no return. They are already overwhelmed, without me needing to slap a stack of Berklee books in front of them. Even the ordinary aspects of living, of social interaction, the things they breezed through before the symptoms hit—none of it goes right, it's all awkward. It's like learning to play with your thumb behind the neck.

The situation is no longer "elective," if it ever had been. A superficial therapy concerned with the "perfecting of neuroses" (as Karen Horney once put it) will only delay the reckoning. The press of desperate circumstance, be it external, internal, or both, dictates that the old adaptation must go— baby, bath water, and all. One hopes to get the baby back later: the creativity within the addiction, the instinctual joy within the sexual compulsion, the healthy self-assertion within the abusiveness, etc. But they're all too admixed, at present, to sort out. Drastic measures are necessary to avert disaster; the sorting will have to wait. I tell my trainees, for the sake of argument, that therapy doesn't change people—events change people. It is the chancy task of therapy to help them survive these events and put them to the best possible use.

I remind my patients that I had the option of not learning to play jazz guitar, but their situation offers no such option. When it's your life (or my life) at stake, there really is no option. Here are the scales.

S N O W   W H I T E

Time and again I have seen malevolent relational distortions in blended families where one parent is impaired and the other, an opportunistic interloper. This is an attempt to apply archetypal thinking as a way of understanding these families and how the children are affected. It appeared in the September 1998 *Psychiatric Times* prefaced with the following disclaimer, which bears repeating:

"As I share a close friend's joy at launching his stepdaughter off to college, I wish to emphasize to my readers that the following exploration in no way generalizes to the majority of stepparents, who, like him, have done their job lovingly and well."

Looking back on their shared childhood with thirty-year-old eyes, my patient admits that what his two younger sisters have recently revealed to him is so plausible as to seem self-evident. It casts a clarifying light on remembered facts: how the girls got rides and sweets from stepdad and he, only chores. How mother would knit alone on the porch late into the night. How, as a ten-year-old, my patient had always felt—almost literally smelled—that something he couldn't quite grasp was wrong about the flow of affection within the family.

So the trip to stepfather's funeral in another state ended up as a relief of sorts rather than one more ambivalent duty. This had been a man who responded to his stepson's sadness about missing his own father by forcibly taking the boy to the cemetery to look at his father's grave and driving away. My patient was left to walk home. Learning the sad fact that this same step-father had sexually abused his sisters at least left my patient in their compa-ny, no longer alone in his sense of having been willfully damaged. He now has a shared reality; a place to start, and my office to sit in while he makes that start.

A fifteen-year-old patient at my rural mental health clinic is not so lucky. Found "parking" with a boyfriend by her widowed father's fiancée, she created an angry scene on arriving home. Her de facto "stepmother" responded by throwing her prom dress, the fruit of many nights' babysitting jobs, into the woodstove.

This episode, the most recent and dramatic of a long series, precipitated a suicide attempt, and after a brief hospitalization whose chief outcome was Depakote, I am expected to add something to the proceedings: another drug, perhaps, or a different DSM label. [Depakote has replaced lithium as the most prescribed treatment for manic-depressive illness; the diagnosis of that entity has expanded so much that almost all extreme or erratic behavior can, for lack of a better explanation, be ascribed to it, i.e. "If all you have is a hammer, all problems are nails."]

The case workers will be orchestrating vigorous family therapy with the goal of reuniting the girl with her father and his new spouse (temporarily, the patient has been farmed out to an elderly aunt). As I listen to their plans and the patient's story and recall the thirty-year-old man in my private office the week before, something tells me this is not going to fly; family therapy and Depakote here are like spitting into the wind. I find these stories merging with a career's worth of similar ones and beyond this composite generic account the outlines of a fairy tale.

In my generic case history, the patient's remaining biological parent is either bereaved or has been abandoned by the other parent. This loss (suffered by a person whose adjustment may have been precarious to begin with) results in wholesale impairment, whether due to psychiatric illness such as chronic depression; to physical injury and chronic pain; to alcohol or substance dependence; or even to just simple incompetence in matters such as cooking meals or opening a bank account, which the other parent may have handled.

Alone in the world, the biological parent pairs up again. The new spouse is an opportunist who enters the arrangement with dubious motivations. This stepfather or stepmother may manage the impaired original parent like a natural resource which produces a paycheck (some are able to marshall enough function to doggedly keep working, but shut down or drink when at home), a disability check, or inherited income. For others, opportunity lies in access to the children: as labor, as targets for the release of anger, or (like the first patient's siblings) as sexual objects. Thus, in varying combinations of neglect and abuse, the children suffer.

How is a clinician to make sense of such ubiquitous, recurring patterns in the lives of his or her patients? The variety of detail in the individual stories, and the complexity of the patterns themselves, make quantification impossible. But somehow they make intuitive sense. Neither medication-oriented psychiatry, with its symptom-suppressing focus, nor the psychoanalytic tradition with its individualistic preoccupation, offer much help. And family systems theory, with which, admittedly, I am ill acquainted, seems entirely too optimistic in bias.

Two psychological traditions look at patterns this large. We will first consult a relative newcomer: evolutionary psychology.

In a recent discussion of stepparenting, the linguist and evolutionary theorist Steven Pinker invokes the universality of the "wicked stepmother/stepfather" motif in folk tales from the Canadian Arctic to Europe to Indonesia—and ethnographic data such as the sanctioned killing of a new wife's prior children among certain aboriginal tribes— to insist that this story is biologically determined. He cites research to the effect that

> "...stepparenthood is the strongest risk factor for child abuse ever identified. In the case of the worst abuse, homicide, a stepparent is forty to a hundred times more likely than a biological parent to kill a young child, even when confounding factors—poverty, the mother's age, the traits of people who tend to remarry—are taken into account."

Pinker's explanation makes sense, as far as it goes: Biological parents are "hard-wired" by evolution to make endless sacrifices only for the offspring that carry their own genetic material forward. (Adoptive parents, unlike the stepparents here discussed, have made a conscious choice to sacrifice.) Yet his conclusion is too weak to sustain the mythic motif of the cruel stepparent:

> "The indifference, even antagonism, of stepparents to stepchildren is simply the standard reaction of a human to another human. It is the endless patience and generosity of a biological parent that is special." [*How the Mind Works*, p. 434]

"Stepparents," he tells us, "are surely no more cruel than anyone else."

Pinker's statement, of course, is true in the general case. Indeed, most clinicians have known stepparents who have been among the best parents in any category, biological included. But the particular stepparents who inhabit the folk tales and cases such as the ones described above present an undeniably concrete reality. This reality goes far beyond Pinker's "standard reaction of a human to another human" into the realm of deliberate and pointed assault on the identity of the stepchild. It is not mere indifference experienced as cruelty, not just magnified memories of ordinary unkindness. These stepparents aim to destroy.

Another discipline that addresses the recurring patterns in the stories our patients relate is that of archetypal psychology, a strand of the Jungian tradition. Instead of the empirical premises upon which both psychoanalysis and biological psychiatry are founded, the archetypal or Platonic view holds that, in an important sense, "fiction is truer than reality." As classically described by Plato himself, we in the world observe only shadows on the wall of a cave, while the figures outside which cast these shadows are "the real thing." Or, in my own favorite example, the *idea* of a Whirlpool is "realer" than its local embodiment in any number of observable whirlpools. We learn about Reality indirectly. Thus, the condensed, dream-like imagery of a fairy tale can help me better understand the particular cases described at the outset, by illuminating the archetypal pattern behind them. No exotic tale is necessary; we need look no farther than the familiar story of Snow White.

> "Mirror, mirror on the wall
> Who in this realm is the fairest of all?"

Just what, exactly, is the "beauty" of which the stepmother/queen, who four times attempts to murder her stepdaughter, is so jealous? What is so lacking in the reflection this mature woman sees of herself in the mirror? Surely the physical beauty of seven-year-old Snow White cannot by itself threaten the grown-up queen so deeply.

The tale opens with anatomical imagery. Snow White's pregnant mother pricks herself with a needle, and her blood on the white snow prefigures the redness of her unborn daughter's lips. Then, years later (mother having died in childbirth), the jealous stepmother instructs her hunter-assassin to bring back Snow White's vital organs as proof of her death. The hunter lets Snow White flee and substitutes the organ(s) of a wild boar (the heart in children's versions; the liver and lungs in the original collected by the Grimm brothers). And the queen, temporarily fooled, has them boiled in salt and eats them.

Snow White is thus twice linked to something vital that is inside (blood, organs) coming out, or being "expressed" in the surgical sense of the word. The queen attempts to replace what is lacking in the mirror—vitality—by ingesting what she thinks is Snow White's own.

The freedom to express what is inside, as opposed to the domination of others and of the weaker parts of the self, is the basis of true psychological autonomy as defined by the Swiss analyst Arno Gruen. "Access to life-affirming emotions, to feelings of joy, sorrow, pain—in short, to a sense of being truly alive—is essential for the development of autonomy as I understand it." The liberty children naturally take to laugh or cry, to show delight or helplessness or need—this is the beauty of which the queen is so jealous; the innocence that she hates.

For her second and third attempts at murder, a disguised (i.e., introjected?) queen overcomes Snow White's suspicion and the warning of the seven dwarves by inviting her to express her feminine beauty (the suffocating stay-lace and the poisoned comb). The final ruse, a poisoned apple, reprises the fruit by which autonomous curiosity was the biblical Eve's downfall.

Why does the stepmother/queen, whether in real or in internalized form, hate the stepchild's innocent autonomy so much? Gruen posits that abusive adults were punished for their own expressions of joy or need as children. To survive psychologically, they may have managed to split off the experience from consciousness. (Faithful to Gruen's larger argument, I here add my own words to a discussion focused on helplessness.) "For the split to be sustained, helplessness [or innocent delight] must become an object of ridicule and hatred ... people will continue to seek revenge on everything that might recall their own helplessness [or the smothering of their joy]."

For the opportunistic stepparents in these clinical cases, the act of exploiting the impaired biological parent, or the stepchildren themselves, may bring this split close to the surface by awakening the stepparents' residual empathy. Such a stirring of human feeling jeopardizes the psychic equilibrium in which their own helpless core lies, long buried; their innocent spontaneity, moribund. A stepchild inhabiting this volatile situation becomes a target. The biological parent offers little more protection than the barely mentioned fairy-tale king.

It is the recognition and devotion of the deep forest's dwarves and finally of a passing Prince from another country that redeem Snow White in the end. Help is not forthcoming from within the family. And though my role in the case of the girl with the burned prom dress is peripheral, and I do not want to cast my jaded rain on the idealistic young case workers' parade, I feel that my position as the psychiatrist carries with it a certain obligation. So I remind them of Snow White's story, not to tell them to abandon their plans for "family reintegration," but to help them appreciate the archetypal forces they are fighting against in pursuing such a goal.

In its typical pop-psychology form, the archetypal approach inevitably lends itself to therapeutic fantasies of integration or individuation. Such resolutions are as oversimplified as the notion that fairy tales have happy endings. In the Grimms' "Snow White," a fantasy of triumphant revenge wins out over any mythic image of wholeness or reconciliation that might be implied by the setting of a wedding party. I have sometimes seen such fantasies endure far into the adult lives of patients.

Iron slippers have been heated over a fire in expectation of the stepmother/queen's arrival. "They were brought over to her with tongs. Finally, she had to put on the red-hot slippers and dance until she fell down dead." In devising such a fate, wherein dance, a self-expressive act, is rendered painfully fatal, Snow White makes a punishment which fits her stepmother's crime.

Raffaela Lamberti Genova
Avelino, Italy ca. 1915

RAFFAELA'S HUG

Published in the *Psychiatric Times* in February 1997 as "Looking for Raffaela's Hug," this piece was intended to be the afterword to my book, *The Helper's Dilemma*, which is devoted to the evolutionary/genetic theory of "reciprocal altruism" and its implications for psychotherapy. I never sold the book to anyone, but I love this essay just the same.

"Raffaela" takes the Tragic view of our therapeutic enterprise, looking at the inevitable limitations of professionalized dyadic helping in our modern, mass culture.

When therapists gather for social occasions, there is generally much more hugging than I can comfortably endure. I have taught myself not to cringe, but would-be huggers no doubt find my response unrewarding most of the time. Nonetheless, I know that I would not even be present at such gatherings if there were not, somewhere within me, a big, fleshy, olive-oil-and-anisette-scented hug that I want to give to the world. It is the hug I got from my grandmother, Raffaela Lamberti Genova.

I am told that Raffaela—it's a pleasure to say her name, for I only ever knew her as "Grandma Genova"—once declared that I was destined to become either a doctor or a priest. As a psychiatrist/psychotherapist I foolishly cast myself as both and sometimes ended up hamstrung in a ridiculously ineffectual arithmetic average of the two, neither fish nor fowl, as the saying goes. Having thereby learned a measure of humility, Grandma's words still enjoin me to integrate the scientific and the moral functions in the interest of my own professional survival.

Grandma's conviction was based on the fact that I hugged her back hard; when I saw her arms splay out as I passed under the grapevine into her kitchen, I would throw mine open too. She herself gave freely to any Catholic charity or mission that sent someone to ask for her hard-won

66

money. Above the kitchen table, with its bottomless plate of anisette cookies, was a picture frame filled with haloed figures—a collage of brochures representing her many donations. My longtime analyst/trainer once shared with me her own gloss on this scene when I described it to her. She imagined haloes also on Grandma and on each little anisette cookie. I think she was trying to teach me about the danger my idealizations get me into. But I am sorry; Raffaela Genova and my French-Canadian grandmother, Alma Berthiaume Plamondon, will forever remain exempt from analysis.

I know now that these two were real women with real problems and real shortcomings. I know this intellectually and from my parents. But to me they were incarnations of Unconditional Love whose hugs I can still, if dimly, smell and feel, whose accented English is still one of my deepest musics.

The danger, as it turned out, was not in idealizing them but in idealizing Unconditional Love itself.

Between my grandmothers and the present is a lot of the usual water under the bridge: struggling parents whose frustrations I witnessed (and frequently caused); small-town conformity; Ivy League expectations of "achievement" versus the reality of painful compromise with the hierarchies that rule professional training and practice; learning to manage both my own depressive constitution and my narcissistic escapes from it; marriage and raising children. The openness Grandma had appreciated receded beneath layers of resentment at hurts real and imagined.

I came to the practice of psychotherapy armed with theories and techniques aplenty. But underlying these was (and is) an idealistic fantasy—shared, as I believe, with most of my colleagues across the spectrum of the helping professions—that I could be a healer. I really wanted some safer way to open myself to people and thereby heal them and myself—to get back, through a circuitous complexity that would somehow protect me, to Alma's and Raffaela's hugs.

I have learned that this is impossible. My grandmas were safe; the world is not. (Theories, techniques, or naive trust in the Lord of Process notwithstanding.) Opening one's self has unpredictable results. Sometimes they can be powerfully positive, and like most writers in the field, I have previously written of my successes, adding a few more case histories to the ever-growing literature of therapeutic victory tales that, from Freud onward, has become one of the dominant mythic forms of our age.

But at other times the therapeutic encounter, the attempt to help using "the self as instrument," as some put it, can be extremely damaging. All experienced practitioners have secret memories of disaster or near-disaster which we rarely share—and when we do, we tend to rationalize them away with theories about why this or that person was really untreatable, poorly motivated, etc. And when we hear the regularly surfacing stories of therapists gone astray — sexual liasons, abandonments, personal lives in "inexplicable" disarray—we take care to mentally distance ourselves from any such possibility. Those involved were of a different order than us, sick or needy or grandiose in some more fundamental way, we tell ourselves, ignoring a quieter voice that says, "There but for the grace of God go I."

Less dramatic, but even more deflating, are the instances in which the effort and risk of opening one's self to another's suffering yields no discernable result at all. We strive for a starring, positive role in someone's life only to find ourselves cast in a bit part.

And yet, since our models are based only on success, that is all we dare dwell upon. Many of us present a brave and well-adjusted face to our patients and colleagues while inwardly cycling through loss of faith, then renewal, then back again. Having no systematic way to take a longer view of our failures, we speak vaguely of our individual "burnout" or fatigue without permitting ourselves to question more deeply: Might our failures point to a failure in therapy itself? While the emotional experience of helping and being helped is unquestionably instinctive and healing, might there be something truly flawed, indeed unnatural, about the context in which we attempt to achieve it? I ask the reader to consider what it means that certain distressed individuals elicit our help then promptly get worse, seeming to unravel before our eyes in direct proportion to the intensity of our straightforward, well-intentioned efforts.

The simple contexts wherein "unconditional" love flourishes and heals are rapidly vanishing in our complex, fragmented, information-numbed society. Its real, hidden conditions usually include shared fundamental vocabularies and values and a narrative connection both to the past and to some reasonably secure and predictable future. When Raffaela hugged me, she gave me more than any one isolated person can. Through her, uprooted immigrant though she was, I received the assurance of an entire culture in which people and events were coherently connected, and even tragedy and pain had their place in a larger scheme. Such was the foundational solidity of her embrace.

When open-hearted therapy works, these conditions are at least partially recreated in the private context of a professional relationship—a sort of miniature, dyadic culture with its own language and worldview. This soothing or challenging dyad can be so rewarding to create, such an antidote to modern loneliness, that we often forget it is an artificial relationship within whose structure compassion and concern are commodified no matter how "genuine" we try to be. Thoughtful patients often make the wry observation that it is as if I am their "hired friend," and I find it helpful to acknowledge their accuracy about the bizarre world we live in, where such a contrived situation may be the most nurturing aspect of their lives.

True, the instinctual human emotions of lovingkindness may allow us, however contrived the context, a transient experience of an eternal present which lies beneath the distractions of culture and chronology. But time's distraction is also real, and it seems prudent to remind ourselves that compassion, concern, empathy, and love evolved over time. These traits, comprising what evolutionary biologists term "reciprocal altruism," are (whatever else they may be) the products of natural selection over millennia within small bands of hunter-gatherers who shared most of their DNA sequences in common. Now, in a complex mass culture, we struggle to shoehorn these emotional templates into the social relations of urban consumer capitalism, of which our beloved psychotherapy is itself an artifact.

Some helping professionals, regardless of credentialed discipline, are more thoroughgoing "doctors" than I. They are capable of a more detached interest and seem ever aware that their role in their patients' dramas is often more symbolic than actual. But detachment, be it mystical, scientific, or therapeutic, has never been my strong suit. As soon as I find the energy, I have an irrepressible impulse to enter my patients' lives with my real self and be affected by them, even though I outwardly maintain tighter-than-average formal boundaries. I know I am not alone in this desire for personal contact. In fact, in working with therapists, physicians, nurses, and other professional helpers through the years—many of them suffering from "burnout"—I have yet to find one for whom this impulse is entirely absent.

This is because, in order to be effective helpers like these, we must be operating from an instinctive base. And if we fail to understand the nature of our impulse to help, its origins and its limitations, we will operate blindly and continue to predictably burn out and/or lose our boundaries instead of creating and maintaining the small social groups within which our healing instincts can be most effective. Secretly or openly we will keep looking for Raffaela's "unconditional" hug in all the work we do and never find it.

"I JUST KEEP PLAYING THE SAME NOTE"

This is a Romantic piece, as optimistic and full of faith as I get. But the dream really happened and its message stands. The figure of Miles Davis corresponds, in my own learning process, to the compensatory "Catfish on the Bottom," or to the "Al's Landscaping guy" from "Lacan at Bonus Bagels" (both case histories above). Of course, any mythic paradigm, such as that of the healing dream messenger here, only captures one aspect of the real and often prosaic process of personality change.

This piece appeared in *Voices* in an issue (Fall 1995) devoted to music in psychotherapy.

As a lifelong disciple of the guitar and mandolin, I have played with and learned from some wonderful musicians both known and unknown. Most legendary among those in waking life was Marion Sumner, the "Fiddle King of the South" who had been the lead fiddler with Patsy Cline's touring band. He once told me how he'd stolen Django Reinhardt recordings from the music store as a boy to learn Stephane Grapelli's violin parts. I still have a tape of us playing "Cry Me a River" together.

But dream life is an equal teacher to the dayworld, and there I have jammed with the Gods: John Lennon, B.B. King, the great Manhattan street musicians. And always there was the strain of keeping up, the anxiety beneath the inflation—until I played with Miles Davis, about three years into my second psychotherapy.

There I was, struggling to hold down, in rapid succession, progressions of intricate jazz chords that are the love of my life and bane of my existence. Miles leaned against the wall blowing his trumpet, playful as Puck, effortless. I couldn't keep up. "Miles!" I finally said. "How do you do it? How do you find all those notes?" "I don't know," was his first reply. Then, after thinking a second: "I just keep playing the same note until it turns into all the other notes." These have been my watchwords ever since.

The real Miles, who died not long ago, was a musical sophisticate, a Julliard-trained dentist's son who infiltrated the postwar jazz underworld. On the face of it, his dream statement to me would have better fit an archetypal, illiterate bluesman. But I think my unconscious (or maybe Miles) was speaking from where Miles' music really ended up, and if you listen to "Kind of Blue," for instance, you will hear a languid Puck playing far beyond the realm of theory. This reminds me that my formal education did not deal a death-blow to my ability to improvise in music, therapy, or life.

Miles' words had further consequences. In music itself, I learned to do what I really can do and stop trying to do things someone else can do better. I play old swing tunes. *C'est tout.* They are in my blood, and I can flail through them, bang on the guitar and yell from the bottom of my stomach, without conflict. If I play them, you will hear them and know what they mean. Sure, I can have some fun doing other things, and I do, but those old socky chords are *mine.* As long as I live, they will live.

In my writing—and part of Miles' lesson to me has been to spend more time writing, since it is my best instrument—it's gone the same way. I'm not trying to come up with a grand theory, a new synthesis of anything anymore. It's not what I'm about. I keep making the same few points, mostly Winnicott's points, over and over, hammering on those same few chords in whatever the context. To my mind, there is no lack right now of ways to understand people. The problem is that for so long I just didn't get it. I took Winnicott, for instance, and made his simplicity into an intricate "object relations theory" when all he was really doing was natural history, playing like Puck and Miles the same few notes over and over. Now I try to simplify the message, to sing it loud and hard until it gets through. I don't need to keep reading everything Winnicott ever wrote, and then synthesizing it with everything Bion ever wrote, etc. I will learn more if I go and see some more patients.

"You must be very confused if you have to come and spend this beautiful day listening to me," said Jiddu Krishnamurti, another of my teachers, to a crowd of seekers bent on idealizing him. He, like Winnicott, hammered on a few simple ideas, from all conceivable angles but with no particular order or system. Like Winnicott's papers, all Krishnamurti's books are fundamentally the same. But still we struggle to get it, and now there is a Krishnamurti Foundation and so on. In order to be understood, these ideas must be lived, not just reasoned through. And then it's time to put away the books and the institutes and the "major-dude" heroes and go find our own chords, sing our own songs. That, I believe, is what Krishnamurti, Winnicott, and Miles wanted for us.

I don't worry about changing what's on my business cards anymore. "Psychiatry and Psychotherapy" is good enough for me. My professional identity has to come from me and my music, not external definitions, salable images, logos. I don't worry if I'm going to be holistic enough for one person, intellectual enough for the next, "authentic" enough for the next, medical enough for the next. I just try to meet them halfway. If I can, they will waste less time finding out whether *I'm* really someone who can help them.

Finally, as a therapist, I try to be a rhythm player. The lead part is for the patients, and if you try to teach them to play like you, they will blow it. When they find the dominant note of themselves, help them to hammer on it. If they are struggling to be smart, pretty, insightful, "genuine," successful, the best this or that—it's always in someone else's terms. If instead they just keep hitting that one note, they'll be the one and uniquely best [fill in name here] the world will ever know, and all the other notes will follow.

GETTING TWO (2.0)
PEOPLE INTO THE ROOM

This piece from the November 1999 *Psychiatric Times* is my ironic response to the challenge of setting "quantifiable goals" for relational psychotherapy. More importantly, it makes some serious points about the nature of the therapy relationship and about therapist burnout or (in more recent psychobabble) "compassion fatigue."

A trainer of mine, the late Barry Wood, M.D., often related an anecdote about a patient who was embarking upon an analysis with him. "Do your best!" she said as they agreed to work together at the close of their first meeting. "No," Barry averred. "I'll do the best I can." The distinction he meant to indicate—between being perfect and being human—is one that is learned and re-learned in progressively more subtle ways throughout the course of a therapist's career.

I get headaches from time to time but can count the times I've canceled my therapy hours these seventeen years on the fingers of one hand. Those are the times I couldn't function in any responsible way. But most of the time I work from my headache, knowing I won't be as quick with insights or interpretations, but asking myself instead: What am I seeing, hearing, feeling about this patient from my present (dulled, heavy-lidded) perspective? I might even decide to announce it. "You know, I have a headache today, so I'm not following this story as well as I might be, but your tone of voice (speech rhythm, facial expression, posture...) make me think (feel) A, B or C."

I can't recall a patient ever complaining about this sort of observation as long as they are assured I am indeed paying attention to them. Aside from feeding back a more global impression to them, I am also modeling an acceptance of oneself "as is" rather than a striving for false perfection.

Very occasionally, with well-established patients, I have even admitted to boredom (residents: don't try this at home), when one of them remarked on my expression and inquired as much. "Yes, I am bored", I might say. "I'm concerned about you and sincerely wish you felt better, but at this moment, I *am* bored. This pattern always repeats itself when you come up against (meet, remember, hope for) A, B or C." Patients already know that I respect and, in some way, appreciate them if I am working with them long term. Money can't buy these prerequisites, which are part of my internal assessment of "fit" from the outset. But at this sort of juncture, patients learn that their fee purchases only my attention and skill, not any particular state of mind on my part at any given moment. This places more responsibility on them to listen to themselves and address what they hear.

I am sitting with a psychologist supervisee who feels relatively "burned out" lately (fortunately, we seem to alternate in feeling this way, as today I do not). He presents an interaction that drained him. The supervisee's patient is an isolated workaholic man. Our beloved DSM would place him in Axis I: Dysthymia, and Axis II: Mixed (narcissistic/compulsive) Personality Disorder; he is among the legions of miserable but highly productive people often trivialized as the "worried well." Recurrently he has been frustrated by his inability to negotiate relationships in which he does not hold all the power. Everyone in the patient's emotional world must be, in some sense, an employee, and in recent months it has dawned upon the therapist that he has become one such himself. The therapist's fantasy is that his patient is destined for a heart attack—aside from a reflection of concern and plausible medical intuition, I wonder if this may also be an unconscious wish for liberation from a man whom he consciously likes and values.

After a two-week absence on the patient's part, the psychologist, traversing the waiting room, has a novel experience. His patient looks up, makes full eye contact with a warm smile, and says, "I'm really glad to see you." Taken slightly aback, the therapist genuinely reciprocates. But once the session formally begins, the familiar litany of grievances resumes—what my supervisee calls "thrashing around"—and the eye contact and openness disappears.

The patient's frustration is contagious, and the psychologist senses that aping the supposedly classical ideal of listening, containing, and receptively empathizing is going to sap his own energy, certainly, and possibly waste the patient's time as well (for they have done a lot of this already). As the psychologist calls it (and I would have), it's time for an active intervention. He takes an experiential route: "You keep saying you want contact. I'm here in the room with you! Make contact with me. Ask me a question!"

But other than showing a little irritation, the patient won't bite. The session lurches to an end... and then the psychologist realizes he's forgotten to tell the patient about his own vacation the following week! The patient dismissively denies receiving the prior written coverage information which the therapist habitually hands out weeks in advance.

My supervisee feels awful; doubly so, I think, because here he'd just offered contact, only to be seen as abruptly pulling away. The feeling stuck with him all evening. (And the ostensibly happy ending, an extra appointment eventually scheduled at the patient's request prior to the vacation, didn't completely relieve it.)

It is of such moments, multiplied by the thousands, that "burnout" is made: at least as much as of the obvious crises and cliff-hangers which one more easily defends against by purposefully going into battle-hardened emergency mode.

This is an experienced psychologist who could as easily be supervising me, so our further conversation attempts to deepen our understanding of this interaction rather than devise some "right way" to handle the situation. In the moment, I probably would have done something similar and have had the same feeling afterwards.

Hypothetically, though, in response to the patient's isolative "thrashing," would there have been a way to do less "work," to avoid trying to make something happen? What if the therapist had just commented retrospectively about the pleasant *spontaneous* connection he had felt with the patient in the waiting room? This would have had several virtues: 1) it might have helped the patient to access a connected feeling without having it feel forced upon him, 2) the statement that contact had been enjoyable would leave the door open for more, and 3) no precedent about the therapist "making things happen" *for* the patient would have been set, no promise made for the future. Thus, when the reality of the vacation gaffe intruded later, it might have been less glaring, since the message to the patient would very clearly be "We were in contact, and I enjoyed it" rather than (even if unintentionally) "My mission in life is to make contact with you." This way the therapist ends up with a little less egg on his face.

A full-bore experientialist, on the other hand, might well have seized the waiting-room moment in real time, commenting on the connected feeling right then and there. The risk of going that route is that he could easily have frightened the patient away, psychically or physically.

If you think these subtleties are too rarified to be worth bothering about, remember how tired you can be at the end of a day doing therapy. In cultivating our interpersonal sensitivity as a tool, we make ourselves vulnerable to the microscopic vicissitudes of human needs and our implied promises to meet them.

For argument's sake, the various possible interventions with our isolative, "thrashing" patient are plotted (Figure 1) on two extremely non-standard axes, whose dimensions I will explain. On the X axis, metaphorically of course, the number of people in the room are plotted, with the maximum (and ideal) number, two, at the center. This dimension concerns the degree of freedom of expression available to therapist and patient, as we will discuss further below. In this era of quantifiable goals, I would like to suggest, only half (0.5) in jest, that this dimension provides a universal, measurable goal common to all relational psychotherapies (e.g. psychodynamic, experiential,

Possible Interventions with Patient (see text)

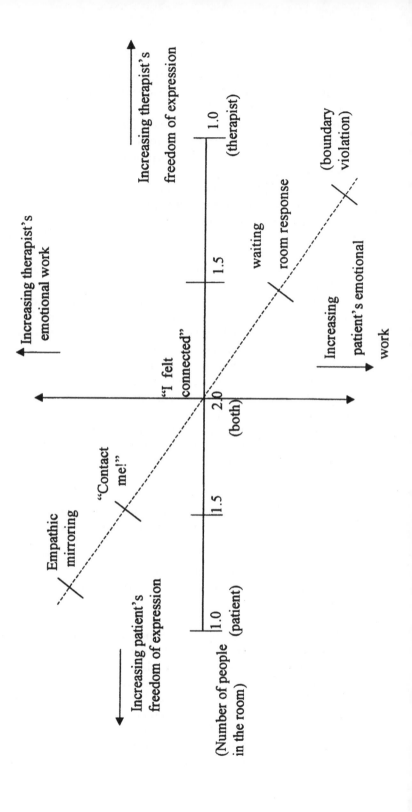

humanistic); that is, to all therapies that are not primarily supportive or directive in nature: to get two (2.0) people into the room.

On the Y axis we have "emotional work," roughly defined as the performance of an emotional function properly belonging to someone else. (The idea of "enabling" from the substance abuse literature is similar, but usually refers to personal, not professional, relationships.) In enacting his patient's frustration about contact with others, my supervisee ("Ask me a question!") was doing the patient's emotional work. The modern popularizer of this concept of emotional labor, Berkeley sociologist Arlie Hochschild, wrote about Delta Airlines flight attendants (their enactment of smiling competence and their private psychic exhaustion) in the early 1980s. We therapists are often emotional wage laborers as surely as Hochschild's stewardesses were.

Let us now survey the entire spectrum of potential interventions my supervisee and I have discussed, from left to right as they appear on the graph. At the extreme left stands an ideal of "mirroring" or receptive empathy and containment. It derives from the neoclassical analytic tradition associated with names such as Winnicott and Kohut (though it may be more a caricature than an accurate portrayal of their clinical work). At the outset, my supervisee was working hard in this mode not to express any personal reactions to his patient's output but instead to respond only in terms derived from that output itself. This effort is shown on the Y axis. In Winnicott's words, contact with the environment at early developmental levels is ideally made "as a part of the life process of the individual" rather than "as a part of the restlessness of the environment." This is not two-person therapy, but what I call "one-person-plus-womb" therapy; there is barely more than one person, the patient, in the room, as the X axis reflects. Without doubt, such an approach can be necessary to establish a beachhead with narcissistically damaged patients.

However, our psychologist wearied of the effort (especially after the suggestive contact in the waiting room) and judged that the alliance was solid enough to risk more of an expression of his real feelings (X axis). So he made the experiential "Ask me a question!" intervention that we have already discussed. At the time, he felt a great relief in (as he described it) "putting the ball in the patient's court." What we appreciated in hindsight together was how much effort (and promise of future effort) this intervention still demanded on the therapist's part (Y axis). There is more of him in the room, but he is still functioning largely as an auxiliary of the patient's. We can count 1.5 people in the room.

Next on the graph comes the hypothetical intervention wherein the therapist would comment sincerely upon his own enjoyment of the waiting-room episode. No promises or injunctions—no strings for either party—are attached to this statement, which implicitly invites the patient to do a little more work (risk-taking) to express deeper feelings more freely. There are now 2.0 people in the room. This situation requires some work from each person, and grants substantial expressive freedom to each in turn.

Furthest to the right we have a second hypothetical intervention. The therapist "seizes the moment" right in the waiting room to comment on the unprecedented connection he feels with the patient. Here the therapist is forgetting how frightening contact is for this particular individual; he has ceased to give his patient's needs adequate respect. This puts an unequal emotional burden onto the patient, who, if he doesn't "flee" (literally or into himself), must try to tolerate vulnerability amidst what feels to him like a threatening intrusion (Y axis).

The X axis reveals that this emotional work from the patient serves the therapist's need for contact; he has "enlarged" himself, thereby pushing some of the patient out of the room. We are down to 1.5 people again, with the majority belonging to the therapist. Going any further to the right on this axis in the direction of serving the therapist's needs would constitute a blatant boundary violation.

To summarize: For each person in the therapeutic dyad, emotional effort—in everyday language, considerateness; in Winnicott's, "contributing-in"—varies inversely with freedom of expression. The goal of the therapy process is not some effortless or perfectly free state of being for either therapist or patient, but instead the "happy medium" of mutual respect and receptiveness that characterizes a healthy working relationship.

As much or more is learned from deviating from, and then repeatedly getting back on, such a course as from managing to stay on it. The latter experience—the occasional interpersonal "click" we have with some patients—is the frosting, not the bread and butter, of our work in individual psychotherapy. If lulled by how good clicking with a patient feels, we may risk missing important information. The experientialists' expectation that therapists should be "energized" by each clinical encounter leads, on an everyday level, to excesses of therapist self-expression and narcissism.

No, an ordinary good-enough collaboration more often feels like work. With time, however, one senses that the repeated corrections in the dynamic balance of two people's emotional effort and self-expression are getting easier and easier. When this occurs, we can be confident that a relational psychotherapy is succeeding. And the better it succeeds, the better prepared our patients will be to fruitfully and autonomously engage with the individuals and groups in their own real lives. Thus, relational psychotherapy is less a solution for their problems than a better start on one.

It is a good thing that patients expect us to do work for them; that's why they come. It is also irreducibly true that we must. In the office and in life, these X and Y axes do not intersect at zero but at two. Nonetheless, the idea that we are there in the office to "help" in some naive way is, in many cases, an expectation well worth frustrating. To cite the pre-pharmacological joke: How many psychiatrists does it take to change a lightbulb? (One, but the lightbulb has to want to change.)

Both by showing patients what they can reasonably expect from another human being and by avoiding emotional exhaustion and so prolonging our own careers, we can often do a lot more by doing less.

THE ENDLESS WALK
OF THE FOOL

The Tarot deck provides an eye-catching image with which to flesh out that hidden grandiosity so often underlying "low self-esteem." The figure of the Fool nicely connects standard conceptualizations of narcissism with the extremely valuable, but less widely known, archetypal perspective of James Hillman.
This piece appeared in the September 1997 *Psychiatric Times.*

Many patients need to render me safer at the beginning of a therapy session. They will try to engage me informally, just as we're entering together and settling in: a comment about the novel on my desk, my new shoes or old shirt, my tan or pallor, fatigue or energy. I typically offer a casual rejoinder and let this go, fearing I would appear stuffy or robotic were I to "call them on it." The fact is, I'd as soon remain safe, also, in this surface realm of friendliness. The depths will appear in due time, and I have a family to support. Social norms today dictate "realness" and caring engagement from the therapist, not the detached procedural stance that prevailed at mid-century.

But a few patients (we will worry about diagnostic categories later) are so persistent in this opening repartee as to make me squirm inwardly and envy those bygone analysts whom custom allowed to keep their own mouths shut. Patients like these will not rest until I let them take care of me in some way— empathizing, complimenting, making me laugh—and then I will owe them something. I will have begun to need them and am thus less likely to destroy them.

I carry this squirminess within me, feeling vaguely unsafe myself in the thrall of their "projective identification," until I find somewhere to use it. This can take several sessions. But just as surely as Winnicott's maxim that a correct but premature interpretation may constitute trauma, an interpretation at the right time provides sweet relief for doctor and patient alike. I can

THE FOOL.

From the Rider-Waite Tarot Deck, copyright US Games Systems, Inc.

at last abandon the eggshell walk of being always kind and never mean. The patient can relax his or her efforts to control me with defensive niceness. A new level of honesty is achieved.

Finding the right time to say something about these particular patients' oppressive friendliness, however, involves listening to their stories for a time. I usually find that they have been trying to do the same thing on a larger scale in other contexts. A man works extra hours at the office to come up with a creative and innovative scheme to show to upper management. The problem is, he wasn't hired to be creative. The Creativity Department has that covered. The boss's indifference devastates him. A woman becomes romantically involved. She regales her new friend with evidence of the intense and passionate soul she really is: offbeat postcards or stormily poetic e-mail messages follow hard on their every date. The boyfriend's indifferent answering machine devastates her.

On the face of it, these patients are victims of that great American epidemic, "low self-esteem." The woman is reaffirmed in her conviction that she's ugly, over the hill (she is quite attractive by any but the most youth-obsessed standards), and stupid (far from it). The man once again finds that he lacks communication skills (he is most articulate) and that elusive, creative spark (I would bet he has more of it than the Creativity Department). Their hurts, endured recurrently, can lead to some awful places: addiction, chronic depressive illness, embittered emotional isolation. Indeed, they may have already led there. So this business of interpretation is no parlor game; the stakes are high. There are times when the concept of a sinking self-esteem, which must be ever buoyed by a "caring," encouraging therapist, is simply the wrong heuristic. Well intended though may it be, this conceptualization tends to throw some patients from our frying pan back into the world's fire. They learn nothing new; we therapists have just let them "win" at their losing game for awhile.

Why do these patients keep getting burned so badly? Because beneath the external "low self-esteem"—here is where interpretation comes in—is a core of grandiosity that can't be touched, that must be preserved at all costs. The woman prefers to believe she is physically or intellectually unattractive in order to hold onto the fantasy that "if only" her love interest could truly see her inner world, the flower that she really is, he could not fail to be won over. The man would rather feel uncreative and inarticulate so he can continue to believe that his sincerity, his earnest enthusiasm could have won his managers' admiration. "If only" is preferable to the more difficult truth that these patients have indeed been seen and not wanted. Not processing this difficult truth, however, keeps a certain naive hope alive. A hope that will likely make them vulnerable again the next time they sense an opportunity and rush to reveal themselves. The pattern can persist until they are thoroughly charred.

Turning to diagnostics for a moment, what we are seeing here is a variant of pathological narcissism. The DSM-IV narcissistic personality disorder category does not capture this variety, focusing as it does on the more obvious arrogant, manipulative and unempathic type who is compensating for the "low self-esteem" hidden inside. Here it is the grandiosity, the irrepressible conviction that imagining something well enough will make it so, that is hidden, as is the subtle manipulativeness beneath overtly empathic behavior (e.g., the patient who inquires about my tired look).

These variations are as two sides of a coin, another expression of "the necessary polarity inherent in every self-regulating system," as Jung described our psyches. The dynamic interplay between them is part of what the DSM categorical disease model misses (although the extremes of "stuckness" in the above two examples could certainly qualify as illness). We are dealing with a narcissistic dimension of personality possessed in varying degrees by most of us and important in the etiology and course of a wide variety of psychiatric and medical disorders.

Analytic developmental theorists traditionally locate the origins of narcissistic disorders in infancy and early childhood, when a "True" (Winnicott) or "Real" (Kohut) Self is invalidated, ignored, or inconsistently recognized by caregivers. Most relevant to the origin of persistent fantasies of omnipotence may be the "warm and cold" situation Winnicott poignantly described, wherein a mother has been "not only not good enough...but good and bad in a tantalizingly irregular manner," recurrently raising, then dashing, the True Self's hope for recognition.

But whatever their origin, these unstable self-concepts are most obvious in association with a later developmental phase: adolescence, when physical maturity lends its power to the demand for recognition. Inquiring historically about this phase, I often get responses like: "Adolescence? I didn't have an adolescence!" which may refer either to parental overprotectiveness or to a premature exposure to adult responsibilities. In either case, one better understands the ongoing adolescent striving in these patients' lives, sometimes charming, sometimes irritatingly insistent.

For these reasons, the Jungian literature on *Puer*, the archetype of the Eternal Youth, provides a more comprehensive metaphor with which to approach these "narcissistically damaged" individuals. One well-known characterization is James Hillman's:

> "The term [*puer aeternus*] comes from Latin epithets for heroic and divine figures. Some mythic figures bearing typical puer traits are...Adonis, Icarus, Jason. But there are puer aspects as well in Horus, in Dionysus, in Hermes, in Jesus. Students of literature would find the puer perhaps in St.-Exupery, in Shelley, Rimbaud...Melville has at least five such beautiful sailor-wanderers....
>
> "In our pathological lives the puer aeternus appears as a specific style of prolonged adolescence, lasting sometimes until 40—and sometimes ending with sudden violent

death." [*Loose Ends*, p.57]

Puer aeternus is a "structure of consciousness and pattern of behavior that struggles with… time, work, order, limits" and "is driven… to inquire, quest, chase… transgress all limits."

In contemporary culture, *Puer* is a dangerously dominant archetype that distorts and often destroys lives of celebrities and artists who become "identified" with it, unwitting vehicles for a whole society's frustrated longing for individual recognition (F. Scott Fitzgerald, Marilyn Monroe, Jimi Hendrix, John Belushi, Kurt Cobain, and so on ad infinitum).

That ancient compendium of Western esoterica, the Tarot deck, wonderfully illustrates this pattern in the figure of "The Fool" (see illustration) who gaily walks off a cliff, his dog jumping at his heels (a warning? or a push?). The Fool is brimful of talent, energy, creativity, but short on follow-through, and he expects the world to fall in line with his schemes. As the Joker, the Fool is the only one of the spiritually potent "'major arcana" to survive in our modern gaming deck. But unlike his mischievous descendant, the original Fool seems to take himself entirely seriously.

When I do find an opening to comment on my patients' unwitting assumption that if they imagine or express something well enough they will make it so, I try to remember the trick is for them to lose the omnipotence—to be "ordinary"—without losing the sense of personal value and uniqueness. Bringing up my own feeling of being coerced by their friendly or solicitous words at the start of sessions, I might remark that other people could react the same way; others who might well find much to appreciate about this person, if given the time.

Occasionally I have taken the risk of sharing an episode from my own adolescence. At sixteen, after a girlfriend had decided she'd had enough of me, I wrote her daily for several months, each missive more soul-baring than its predecessor. Our long driveway led uphill to the mailbox, making my heart beat even more rapidly as I walked there, anticipating a response. How could she refuse these beautiful pleas? But the mailbox always clunked hollowly. Eventually I gave up; when or how, I don't remember.

It is tempting to say that when I understood that my omnipotent fantasy had to die, the rest of me could get on with living. But this is just a more refined version of the same fantasy, one which substitutes the "mature" faculty of intellectual understanding (for Jungians, *Senex*) for youthful imagination. Neither is all-powerful; neither our personal worth and talent, nor our intellects, can guarantee recognition, love, happy endings, or freedom from pain and rejection. Understanding and interpretation cannot stop the Fool from going to the mailbox. His walk is endless. Even those who have been blessed with outward recognition attest to this.

In sharing my walk with patients, I am only trying to help shift this vital and necessary psychological principle towards a place where it can inspire, rather than dominate, our lives.

ROCKABYE BABY:
WINNICOTT'S HATRED

Anyone who has read this far is aware of how deeply D.W. Winnicott's work has affected me. This is my declaration of independence from him. It was published as the companion piece to a re-publication of his famous mid-century paper "Hate in the Countertransference" (which had appeared in *Voices* in the 1950s) in a "Best of" issue to finish out the millennium, Winter 1999. If you haven't read Winnicott's paper, you should; it can also be found in his first book, *Collected Papers: Through Paediatrics to Psychoanalysis* (1958). In *Voices* I prefaced the master's paper with the following introduction:

"In reading Winnicott's classic, younger readers should be aware that his 1949 categories of 'psychosis' and 'schizophrenia' were far broader than those of the present day. Many of us now find these ideas most useful for understanding the spectrum of developmentally trauma-tized personalities, regardless of diagnostic category."

Why have I always avoided a thorough reading of this paper? I knew of it, glanced at it several times. This must be a symptom of something because for years Winnicott was the only writer who made sense to me. I read a good part of his entire output, taught courses, and even gave an AAP Summer Workshop presentation on him (1992). What was this avoidance about?

Reading the paper now, I see that its ambivalence stands at the heart of an impasse I couldn't get through in my own primary psychotherapy—five years with the woman who, more than anyone else, trained me and contin-ues to influence my work. Our impasse, I believe, exemplifies a more gener-al problem: What are therapists and patients to do with hatred, the long shadow cast by this strange business of professionalized loving?

Because I couldn't get my therapist to admit her hate for me, I could never feel fully accepted and loved by her. (Winnicott: "If the patient seeks objective or justified hate he must be able to reach it, else he cannot feel he can reach objective love.")

I brought my therapist much need, and much resentment; I would express self-righteous proletarian rage at her material privilege and apparent glowing health. How she must have hated me! For, as I later found out, she had been undergoing a series of demoralizing surgical procedures attempting to treat her infertility (I imagined that her absences were lecture tours), and that, stressed by the inability to have children, her seemingly magazine-perfect marriage was failing. But, embodying the other pole of Winnicott's own ambivalence, she felt it was her role to "therapeutically" contain her hate. (Winnicott: "A mother has to be able to tolerate hating her baby without doing anything about it. She cannot express it to him.")

Lord knows I kept trying. When neither mocking nor insulting her, nor bringing in dreams of her as a demon/witch, budged her from her deeply caring stance, I would bring her reading. Like the Holocaust philosopher Jean Amery's essay on torture. Or listening. Like Richard Thompson's ballad of abandonment, "Down Where the Drunkards Roll."

Being human, of course, she did leak. Once I recall her "tangentially" citing Winnicott's list of reasons for mothers to hate their babies (it comes from this paper—another clue to my avoidance?). And once, early on before she'd become entirely consistent in her stance with me, I remember this diminutive Jewish woman suddenly becoming a fundamentalist preacher as she forcefully mirrored back my endless complaints about her wealth and status: "It's like you're begging me, Paul, OPEN UP THE PEARLY GATES! OPEN UP THOSE PEARLY GATES!" For a moment, I saw myself clearly. That was a tearful ride home that day.

But she did care for me deeply, and had sufficient emotional reserves so that she wasn't forced to inhabit Winnicott's paradox that "love includes hate", as real 24-hour mothers must. (Years later she opines that a childless woman's maternal instinct, plus a therapist's sense that she should be providing unconditional love, were an unfortunate combination.)

And perhaps she somehow judged that I was too fragile to withstand any expression of her hatred. Was I? I will never know.

So as time went on, my therapist stayed in treatment mode, curious about the transference, offering empathy and rigorous dream interpretation—the long-term, midwife-the-innate-healing-process fix—with occasional well-meaning intrusions of more obvious mechanical fixes, like suggestions about homeopathy. The latter were easier to identify and rage against.

We stayed stuck. With her unable to "own," or maybe even consciously feel, the hate I sought in her, I had to leave therapy, expressing whatever hate I could tolerate by firing her. The sporadic (and still professional) relationship we have had since works much better, because as two human beings we can now enjoy, respect, and (to employ a later Winnicottian term) "use" one another. But for me there remains a wedge of doubt, and I know I am kin to Winnicott when he speaks of his own practice as "an attempt on the part of the analyst to carry the work of his own analysis further than ... his own analyst could get him."

Many have seen in Winnicott a new kind of therapeutic heroism as he holds Margaret Little's hand in silence, session after session (see her *Psychotic Anxieties and Containment*). Appreciative of his sacrifice, which was curative in Little's case, I also see it in a perversion of our genetically based primate altruism which evolved not in dyads but in reciprocal social groups over millennia in our common African homeland. For most patients today, finding or making a functional group is a much safer bet than finding a Winnicott who has unlimited time and not much else to think about. Individual depth therapy as we know it, and as some of us (myself included) still practice it, has its place—but not as a reigning ideal. Helping patients to better "use" the real individuals and groups in their lives is of no less potentially transformative value.

Winnicott's legacy for our profession is, above all, his ambivalence, poignantly described in this paper, about containing versus expressing hatred as a caregiver. Despite the friendly rhetoric about being just "good enough," despite his own humble self-presentation, his theory implies either 1) a virtuoso therapist ideal wherein perfect timing resolves the love/hate paradox inherent in professional care or 2) faith in some Greater Good-Enough which guides the therapist in such matters of timing and of expression vs. containment. Real individuals, even gifted therapists like mine, cannot reliably live up to these ideals, because one human being is *too much* for one other human being—whether good enough, perfect, perfectly imperfect—to *reliably* care for or carry faith for. Thus, Winnicott's noble example (like the best of our own experiences as therapists) distracts us from the urgent need to heal societies, communities, families; to stop overloading the relational Dyad, stop trying to defy our emotional biology.

In engendering his modern, individualistic myth of the therapist-hero, Winnicott asks those social primates who are psychotherapists to become gods on a routine and purchasable basis. We are to carry and contain the inevitable hatred which arises in an isolated and easily overwhelmed helper, then express it only at the right-enough time and in the right-enough amount, all the while deftly surviving the hatefulness of our patients. Such is the dubious gift of one of the most influential therapists of all time. He has left us to carry his hatred. Much as I love him, I hate him for that.

Our Trainees' Calling, Our Job Description

In a chapter on the psychotherapy training of novice psychiatrists, Jim Gustafson contrasts two types: "the attuned who lack perspective" and "the discerning who lack empathy." Each has something different to learn. This supervisee was in the former category. But her attunement seemed to go beyond the personal level and needed to be understood and named as "spiritual"—much as I try to avoid that overused word and nebulous concept whenever I can. This piece appeared in *Psychiatric Times* as "Our Residents' Calling..." in February 1996, and almost simultaneously in the Winter 1996 *Voices* with the more general "Trainee" title and language.

My new supervisee freely admitted that she found psychodynamics hard to take seriously. She was not widely read in the analytic classics, but she did assert her conviction that there are lessons to be had in pain and suffering, which seemed as reliable a point of departure as any.

Upon returning to the senior residency year after a long maternity leave, she had been pleasantly surprised to find that a number of her former therapy patients had called anticipating her arrival, wanting to resume. So central was the new child to her present emotional life that she honestly didn't know if she had it in her. "My feelings are so strong for this baby that I'm dreaming all the time just to have time to feel them all," she told me.

In taped therapy sessions her verbal interventions often seemed tentative and inconsistent. Intellectually she had a way of quickly spinning, then equally rapidly discarding, hypotheses. In one notable instance she asked her patient an insensitive question, which in my own hands would have been a blunder and quite possibly the end of the therapy. Yet the relationship was hardly ruffled—in fact it audibly deepened and her patient attended faithfully. My own experience of being with this resident was parallel: Though she was superficially somewhat awkward, she conveyed an underlying self-assurance that made me feel comfortable, even soothed. She had been an internist but found that her patients' physical illnesses often reflected their problematic lives, and she had wanted more time to talk to them.

This resident's aptitude for healing seemed to operate at a very deep level. I felt myself in the presence of a woman of superior spiritual power. (I will postpone definitions for the moment.) Wary of my own capacity for projection, I contained this feeling for a few weeks and scrutinized it. She was part Mexican, and though she knew of no Indian ancestry, her features for me had a distinctly Native American cast. Perhaps this had evoked my fantasy of the *shaman*.

I continued to be somewhat frustrated in my attempts to help my supervisee find a coherent approach to psychotherapy theory and technique... and most of her patients continued to progress. Thinking that her innate aptitude might be generating a subtle resistance to my offerings, I decided to speak openly about my impressions of her by way of more specifically framing my "job description" as her supervisor. With trepidation I told her that I thought she had a spiritual gift: a special capacity to be with another human being in pain; a thirst for, and an ability to remain intact in, the depths. She was surprised and flattered but did not dismiss this acknowledgement. Rather, she seemed to recognize herself in it. It put something into words for her that modesty (and perhaps anxiety) had prevented her from stating overtly to herself.

This done, I told her that her contacts with patients were liable to be haphazard unless she learned some of what I wanted to teach her. Her gifts could reach a wider range of patients than those with whom she happened to fit well from the start. My job would be to better acquaint her with the "middle depths" of individual psychology: the rocks and shoals of cognition polarized by emotion, transference, and defense mechanisms. In this shallow water she would do well to supplement her intuition with both a rough-and-ready developmental theory and a way of thinking about adaptation to temperament.

My acknowledgement had a freeing effect on our supervision process. Her gift had been seen and placed on a different level from psychology rather than remaining its covert competitor. This allowed her to become interested in psychodynamics, and her technical flexibility increased. I don't know whether she will choose (or even have the option) to become an analytically oriented long-term therapist, but the kinds of questions she has learned to ask should help her work more successfully with her patients in whatever context she finds.

Surveys indicate that this particular trainee has two attributes in common with many of the residents now entering psychiatry. She is joining us in mid-career from another medical specialty. And she is attracted by the opportunity to practice psychotherapy despite its contemporary eclipse. This group is important to the immediate future of our stigmatized, uncertain field. They are clinicians, not neuroscientists, and though they may gratefully welcome whatever help medical technology has to offer, they are drawn toward intimate contact with suffering people. What brings them here?

In psychiatry we have a lingering tradition, inherited from analysis, of looking at this thirst for the depths as pathology. The typical formulation casts the future therapist as the child of a depressed or otherwise needy mother. He (or she) becomes exquisitely attuned to mother's emotional messages as a matter of his own survival—sometimes even literal survival. Only to the extent that he is able to meet mother's needs, some of his own may secondarily be met by her. From this early narcissistic distortion, a fantasy of self as omnipotent healer derives which later draws the adult into an "impossible profession" whose structure (regardless of espoused ideology) makes him responsible for the emotional state of the Other.

Within this tradition, the new practitioner may trace these developments in his own training psychotherapy and may then choose to carry on with his motivations more conscious and therefore less dangerous. But accurate as the pathologic formulation may be, it seems we have nothing more positive to say to him (or her), nothing akin to the idea of celebrating a "calling" to the ministry or priesthood with its attendant mechanisms for the evaluation of "spiritual fitness."

In a discussion of "complex idealists," among whom I would include this group of trainees, James Gustafson makes a blunt and accurate statement. "We never talk about spirit in psychiatry. It is even strange to place spirit and psychiatry in the same sentence. We feel their repulsion of each other." [Dilemmas, p.124.] And so I come reluctantly to attempt a definition where the dictionary is of little use.

The spiritual person, for me, is one who has a subjective experience of him/herself, and of others, as being the embodiment of a larger Life Force or Flow. Someone like my supervisee has this experience strongly and consistently enough to ground her interpersonal interactions in it—this is what I meant by her power. Some of the rest of us have rare flickering glimpses of such an experience. For still others I am sure this paragraph makes no sense at all.

Spiritual physicians tend to be fascinated by the human capacity to endure suffering and feel privileged to share the triumph of survival and the solemn mystery of surrender. These are joys and sorrows common to much of medicine, but in traditional primary care (in which I include psychiatry), the patient, and we ourselves, become part of a visible story. This, I submit, is what continues to attract a substantial number of our residents.

I would expect this conception to elicit certain predictable reactions. Scientific positivists will find it irrational, based as it is on subjectivity. Some others of an analytical mind will smell a defense mechanism pitted against a meaningless, atomistic reality. To these I have no defensible answer and can only say, maybe so.

Two other critiques are of more interest to me because they seem to comprehend the intensity of spiritual experience. One is that of social constructionism, as presented by Philip Cushman, an historian of American psychotherapy. To him, what we call Spirit is a "cultural artifact"—a societally determined "enchanted interior" of boundless plenty which mirrors the outward ambitions of the isolated striving self in our late-capitalist consumer society. Opium of the masses, 90210. (The Tibetan Buddhist Chogyam Trungpa once made the same observation about much American "spirituality.") This bears watching. The cult of the Collective Unconscious is every bit as "virtual" as the World Wide Web and can divert us from making real communities and effecting urgent social change.

Yet when I return to my work with patients, or to ancient scriptures and timeless works of art, I cannot reconcile myself to the idea that there are no universals, only cultural texts. Repeating themes are everywhere in the human drama. This the Jungian analyst James Hillman appreciates. In his classic 1979 essay "Peaks and Vales" he makes much of the distinction between spirit (Greek *pneuma*) and soul (*psyche*) by way of exploring the contemporary confusion between psychotherapy and spiritual practice. (The early Church decided to make the two terms synonymous, to the everlasting detriment of Western culture as far as Hillman is concerned.)

Spirit is associated with archetypal ideals such as unity, growth, and wholeness which we mortals strive to capture by climbing to the ecstatic heights (cf. Maslow's "peak experience") or plunging to the profound depths. For us limited flesh-and-blood humans, these godly domains may swell our egos and tempt our wills to escape the world's fetters. Such inflation or possession can be both isolating and disastrous.

Soul, by contrast, travels mortal through the earthly "valley of the shadow of death." Its existence is its pathology; an expression of myriad little details of time and place. The cultivation of soul—which for Hillman is the proper role of *psycho*therapy —leads to both humility and humor. It must involve "History, the Great Repressed," both individual and cultural. My efforts with my supervisee attempted to acquaint her with the mundane geography of this middle domain.

Even if present trends intensify and psychiatry persists primarily as a mechanistic trade, trainees of this type will still be drawn to the field for its irreducibly human side. If we do nothing but diagnose these trainees' narcissistic injury, if we offer them no spiritual sustenance, they will have to look for it outside the profession. They may slip away to weekend retreats or New Age bookstores or, if they are very lucky, maintain a positive connection to some valued religious tradition they grew up with. They may learn bodywork, homeopathy, or meditation on their own time. But they will carry within them an unfortunate split between Spirit and the day-to-day business of medical psychiatry, and this will weaken the integrative potential of both their work with patients and the development of the field.

My plea is not for trainers to become something we may not ourselves be, nor for psychiatry to encompass Spirit as such. Rather, I want us to retain, develop, and teach our own soul tradition, as exemplified by Jung, Winnicott, and many others. Their psychologies of meaning at least open onto the depths. Nurtured in this tradition, these trainees will not simply inhabit but flourish within and contribute to our medical discipline.

PART III:
THE PSYCHIATRIC
PERSUASION

INTRODUCTION TO PART III

A pithy observation is attributed to the New York psychiatrist Robert Michels. He quipped that our profession has gone "from the brainless psychiatry of the 1950s to the mindless psychiatry of the 1990s." Why then do I include this last set of essays, originally addressed to psychiatrists, in a collection on psychotherapy?

Psychiatry has indeed decentered from psychotherapy, both from the intellectual dominance of psychoanalytic theory and from an everyday focus on human relationships. Economic forces have shifted our view from the treatment of individuals to the treatment of "populations" and from unique to standardized forms of therapy.

New medications have given us the power to rapidly and profoundly alter disturbed mental states. As often as not, my own columns in *Psychiatric Times* have appeared beside large advertisements for Prozac, Effexor, Risperdal, or Zyprexa. My fellow *Times* columnist, Peter Kramer, was among the first to publicly notice that some of these medications seem not only to treat disease but to catalyze personality change. Thus, contemporary psychiatrists who remain interested in people and their stories are thrown into a confusion of roles: Should they be therapists or mechanics?

Actually, I have found this to be a useful tension and one that has lessons for non-medical therapists as well.

Because of his or her position in society poised between high-tech and high-touch, and expected to take on all comers, the psychiatrist *must* think integratively to do an adequate job. Sooner or later all therapists, medical or not, have to confront (or willfully ignore) at least three realities that thrust themselves upon psychiatrists from the start.

The first reality I have alluded to already: Biological treatments can help, can even save lives. The mind is indeed hosted by a brain, and manipulation of that brain has given our troubled patients options they never had before. Compassion dictates that we offer them these options, and a new sort of Puritanism counters it and suggests we deny them. Either way we are drawn into playing God; the only choice we have is whether or not to be aware of it. Each patient brings a whole new set of moral and existential questions.

The second reality psychiatrists must face is that of social disadvantage versus privilege. Huge segments of society have no access to the kind of treatment many therapists aspire to provide. Our brand of self-awareness, when made available to these people, may make lives without choice even more painful. The mentally retarded and the chronic psychiatrically ill are often prisoners of a largely symbolic and inarticulate existence. What survives in such people is, in my experience, that which is most essentially human.

A final reality of which we psychiatrists are constantly reminded is that some people are broken and cannot heal. Here our therapeutic fantasies meet their demise, but sometimes a more profound sort of contact between clinician and patient happens in a realm beyond cures and "outcomes."

Whatever the place of psychiatry in the future, and whether or not psychotherapy as I have known it has a role within it, the experiences we have had and the lessons we have learned in these decades were real. If the lessons are forgotten, others will have to learn them again.

WHY I LOVE LEWISTON

This essay has always been among my personal favorites, and it got a lot of responses from psychiatrists around the country engaged in hard, unprestigious, and often thankless work who identified with the feelings expressed here. Lewiston (where I still work in the same clinic) provides a real-world balance to my own private psychotherapy practice; it keeps me honest.

"Lewiston" appeared in the November 1994 *Psychiatric Times*.

Your vacation in Maine is unlikely to include Lewiston, unless you have a child at Bates College or need gas on the way to the mountains. This decaying mill-town of 64,000 is not on any list of sights to see. Here, one day per week I come to write prescriptions at the local public mental health clinic. I look forward to these days and these patients, perking up when I hit the turnpike north. My reasons for loving Lewiston stand not only for this unique place but also for the general potential of work few psychiatrists willingly choose to do—for the rewards and lessons of treating sick patients from an ignored and disenfranchised underclass. We don't claim to be on psychiatry's "cutting edge" here. But we are on its living edge.

Descending exit 13, thirty-five miles from the warring gourmet coffee outlets of Portland, my first stop is for gas-station coffee on Lisbon Street. Eight O'Clock brand. I am not the only one hefting take-out coffee as I cross the clinic parking lot. An addictions purist would sneer at the personal disequilibrium reflected in our need for a stimulant jolt with which to confront the day ahead. But in Lewiston, addictions purists and gourmet coffee are both in short supply.

This smallish place has big-city problems. The high HIV rate parallels the prevalence of intravenous drug use. The proportion of students completing high school is lowest among Maine cities. A young man's cracked-skull tattoo or a young woman's sky-high new perm may be their most prized possessions. People feel small and want to feel bigger.

The predominant population is white, French-Canadian by ancestry, lured here from rural poverty when Quebec lost a third of its population in the last century. They came to live in tenements, work in factories, and worship in cathedrals. The factories closed. Older people speak an odd French heard little in the cities of modern Quebec. English here is clipped but musical, with plural "s" sounds frequently dropped even by people who know only English. On my mother's side, these are my people, and sometimes the racial resemblances in this long-isolated gene pool are startling enough that it seems I'm talking to my own family. An uncle's rueful grin or an aunt's particular compulsiveness were things I accepted as just parts of them before I had clinical eyes. Perhaps I never knew how they suffered.

I plug in my laptop and exchange greetings with the agency therapists. It's okay to be tired; everyone else is. I am computerized (for a false sense of security about drug interactions or calls from private patients), but the agency's medical records are not. A stack of them awaits. Yet I will mourn the day they become electronic. Some tangible reflection of the weight and disorder of patients' lives, the irretrievable losses in them (mocked by the disappearance of lab slips into a vast bulk of meaningless paper), will be replaced by the misleading order of the disk.

I get an update on a patient's condition before the scheduled day starts. Many of the professionals here are longtimers. Despite the policy trend toward "case management" for the severely ill, good long-term therapy still goes on here; I have seen its results. These therapists give of their hearts. The polite rules are freely broken. Therapists give advice (and God help Lewiston if they didn't!). They engage in self-disclosure, but not of the guru-gives-self-as-shining-example variety. It's more like: "When I had my operation ...." They visit patients at home or at new job placements, and are appreciated for it. Yet boundary violations rarely become an issue, and there is a lightness to therapist/patient interactions that does no disrespect to the gravity of patients' problems and is harder to achieve in an upscale private office. The major toll here is on the therapists who persist in risking and caring, eschewing detachment which might protect them more, disappoint them less.

The morning flashes by in twenty-minute segments. I dutifully tear the triplicate prescriptions and put each in its lawful place (white for the patient, yellow for the pocket in the back of the chart, pink for the void). I am more resentful and less reliably obedient about informed consent forms which eat up the time I could use to really explain something and often seem to create a self-fulfilling prophecy of medication side effects.

The high-volume nature of this setting is not negotiable; we all adapt to its shortcomings. "Med visits" are vignettes, some tragic, some uplifting, some conflictual. There is a woman in her mid-forties finally emerging from years of rapid-cycling psychotic hell on an empirical stew of antipsychotics, anticonvulsants, and lithium, newly able to begin grieving the wreckage of her life; a twenty-one-year-old schizophrenic mother, pregnant with number three by her boyfriend in prison, playing unselfconsciously with her bright two-year-old, who is obviously well nurtured against all odds; an exhausted middle-aged man with back pain and depression descending relentlessly into the workers' comp/disability morass, defeating all conceivable interventions; and so on.

Unless dementia or acute psychosis are at issue, I rarely do any formal mental status testing, feeling that if I have twenty minutes I will learn more from listening to how patients relate the events of their recent lives, how they try to reason about them, what they allow themselves to feel about them. But I also listen to renew my doubter's faith; I need recurring, tangible proof that people and relationships can still grow under conditions where survival, not "enrichment," is the problem at hand. I truly enjoy seeing most of these patients and they know it. Appreciating them may be the most curative thing I do.

My office-mate, Larry Salvesen, M.D., has decorated the walls with turbulent seascapes which form an apt backdrop for the morning. One tries to steer between polarities of perception, wary of any model that fits too well. One moment it seems I'm practicing the precise science of psychopharmacology, appropriately applying indicated treatments for syndromes which respond predictably, sometimes miraculously. The next I hear an angry Thomas Szasz in the background and wonder whether I'm just drugging family or societal problems—"spreading mellaril on the waters," as an old teacher once put it. One moment I am thankful to have medication to shore up a patient's ability to cope and blunt the raw edge of her agony, and the next I wonder whether I'm enabling someone's addiction and helping him continue to avoid dealing with his problems. I am sure all of these characterizations apply at one time or another. I offer what I am here to offer and hope for the best. As Lao Tzu says: "Trust the trustworthy...and trust the untrustworthy."

I find it impossible, in this context, to make contact with acutely distressed patients without a willingness to enter a primitive-object world where I cannot predict or control the role I will play. I may appear to be the sage, who understands perfectly, a projected Good Parent bearing the modern equivalent of a magic potion. Or the script may cast me as the Stupid Asshole Doctor, a punitive or neglectful authority figure who peddles brain-poison. Storming out of my office might be the most autonomous thing the patient has done in years.

My price for trying to accept all this with equanimity is that I rarely censor my spontaneous self: its bluntness, its playfulness, its tendency to wonder aloud. Though not without risk, this usually brings the patient and me closer together, as does the effort to shift among many levels of language and social ritual. I see an unemployed laborer one minute; a jazzy young barmaid the next; a thoughtful ex-teacher; a holistic hippie carpenter; a fundamentalist farmer; a mute retarded man who needs a reassuring touch; a combative, demented old lady who calls upon my French for an *asseyez-vous!* or a *soyez tranquil!*

There are always hard bargains to be struck in Lewiston, always the search for compromise and the lesser of evils which might allow a life to keep on limping ahead. One cannot lose sight of the reality of brokenness here as one can in a certain exclusive type of private practice to which patients ostensibly come to "grow" and "explore." With their backs against the wall, patients and therapists in Lewiston grow and explore out of desperation...yet, suprisingly often (maybe more often than the "elective" growth-seekers) they get to something true and valuable. And failing that, brokenness and despair are met as real experiences, with compassion whenever humanly possible.

Chronic patients are often intelligent people saddled with identity-disrupting biological vulnerabilities and immense psychosocial disadvantages. They develop an impressive wisdom when they survive. Wasting no energy on pretense and indirectness, they become (in Oliver Sacks' words) "transparent to their experience." Since most of the people we see here are uneducated and their wisdom largely non-verbal, their attempts at putting it into words often fall into cliches: "I just keep on going," "I can't worry about what people think of me." But, like AA's "first things first," "higher-powered" bumper stickers, these are the words of those who have walked the walk. Their meaning is renewed coming from these mouths.

There are societal lessons here also; some things are not covered in medical school. One learns the truths of our culture's Shadow from those unprotected by material privilege. Class and racial divisions will not be erased by welfare money, liberal good will, and more prisons. There are those that work, those that shirk, and those that learn to play the system. But these people who have to adapt to the world's real prevailing conditions—whether outwardly compliant or overtly enraged, whether attractive, repulsive, manipulative, or frightening—will be the wellsprings of the new, for better or worse. Social policy experts who may mean well, but who think and feel in familiar middle-class categories, will not be the architects of the future. People on the Lisbon Streets of the world will always have surprises for them.

At lunch I cross Lisbon Street and walk up Applesass Hill among the neatly kept residential lawns and through a forgotten bird sanctuary. Here a piliated woodpecker thrived all winter, scattering chips on the snow-covered beer cans, his bobbing red head a reminder of all that flourishes amid decay. On Lewiston's streets one is never far from the watchful eyes of the Virgin Mary—her stone statues abound. Here where incest and rape are endemic and need no hypnotist to elicit their memory, the archetype of a virgin mother has not lost its power. No one is dismayed if I pause to cross myself and quietly recite a Hail Mary that echoes down from childhood. People in Lewiston are not above praying.

A favorite local custom is to half bury a bathtub on end and place the statue in the resulting arched shelter. The Virgin Goddess enclosed by a vessel of transformation: The Jungians would have a field day with this image! I am comforted that there are no Jungians on Applesass Hill. From here on clear days I can see Mount Washington, its snow-capped top like the Virgin's wimpel as she looks down on Lewiston, doing nothing, forgiving everything.

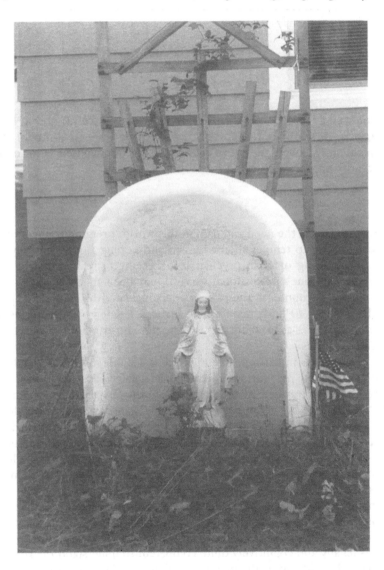

Bathtub Madonna, Lewiston, Maine

TAKE CARE OF HIM

This later clinic tale (*Psychiatric Times*, September 1999) shows how a therapist's developmental perspective informed medical-model work with a severely ill woman, not to "synergize in effectiveness," but only to deepen my appreciation of an inescapable tragedy.

There is no end to the need and pain in this world. I remind trainees of this regularly, trying to temper their idealism and hoping I don't entirely succeed. But growing older in psychiatry forces one to realize that in some important ways one's professional survival may be as much at stake in any given clinical encounter as the patient's personal survival. In middle age we have less energy to burn maintaining elaborate defense mechanisms and images of ourselves as ideal doctors. We learn to husband our resources and choose our battles.

The patient is in her mid-twenties and is a single mother with a history of a prolonged psychotic manic episode. I have seen her a few times before after she transferred to me from another psychiatrist whom, she said, "lectured" to her about her many "high-risk behaviors," whose details I will leave to the reader's imagination. The previous physician had also been understandably uneasy about reducing her dosage of mood stabilizers. Since the patient was willing to stay in treatment, I decided that the lesser risk was to meet her halfway and try to influence her over time. I am still at least that idealistic.

In our first meeting I had established to my own satisfaction that she was no longer psychotic or manic but simply nihilistic. "Life's a crap shoot anyway," she maintained, as I remarked on the chances she continued to take. She was legally and cognitively quite competent to understand the risks she was taking. I could have pathologized her nihilism as "reaction formation" or the "foreshortened future" of post-traumatic stress (a diagnosis for which she also qualified), but not only was her philosophical fortress impregnable, it was an expression of her autonomy and intelligence. Arguing with or diagnosing this bleak vision of life would be an attempt to take these things away, as the first psychiatrist had discovered.

So I established some small alliance with the patient upon a cautious, negotiated reduction in one of the mood stabilizers and an acceptance of her nihilism punctuated by irreverent quips and gallows humor from both sides of the desk. I let her be a bad girl, and I liked her, particularly when I saw how fiercely protective she was of her young son. Predictably enough she decompensated somewhat with the dose reduction. But the case manager was in close contact, and by all accounts the patient continued to function well, finding her emotional struggles a fair trade for "feeling more of what's inside me."

Today, though, the young woman announces triumphantly that she's been off all her medications for two weeks and feels wonderful. From the elation of early mania her retrospective is, "I didn't know how much those drugs were screwing me up!" Gingko biloba and kava kava [popular herbal supplements] will now be entrusted with the treatment of an illness that once needed a three-month hospital stay and bilateral ECT to be brought to heel. [The bilateral procedure is the more powerful type of electroconvulsive therapy, usually reserved these days for more difficult cases.]

"It's not like putting all that junk into my body when I don't know what it is!" she asserts confidently. "These things are natural." (So is arsenic, I stop myself from saying.)

It is not even 10:00 A.M., and a whole rack of clinic patients lies ahead. I care about and like this young woman, but the same can be said of most of the remainder of my schedule. I am one human being. If I were younger, I might let myself get half an hour behind in order to mount a persuasive argument along the following lines (with appropriate adjustment for the low educational level of the patient).

Gingko, kava, and other herbs may be useful substances, but they are not treatments for major psychotic illnesses. (It's not these, but the omega-3 fatty acids [derived from fish or flax oils] that are rumored to be "natural" mood stabilizers, anyway.) Historically, psychoactive herbs were not, as far as I know, maintenance treatments. They were used short-term, in low doses, within a very different social context. In the blasting wind of industrial mass culture, herbs stand little chance of keeping my patient's fragile candle burning quietly; it will either go out or set the house on fire. I do not doubt that my own industrial antidotes, the conventional mood stabilizers lithium and valproate, have caused her significant side effects. But sometimes life drives a hard bargain; chronic illness often demands choosing the lesser of evils.

I could go on to extol the virtues of gabapentin (which probably wouldn't work) or lamotrigine (whose boldface rash warning would ensure that the patient would never take it). [Both of these antisiezure medications are now used as mood stabilizers.] I could tell her that a transient, energized sense of well-being commonly occurs when people stop their psychotropics. That, based on her history, this was likely to yield, sooner or later, to irritability and paranoid psychosis. That some or most of the "side effects" of which she now complained had in fact been symptoms of inadequate levels of medication following the dose decrease.

But the patient's movement now is away from psychiatric care: Her agenda is to defy an authority figure, and I will be her straw man as I deliver yet another "lecture." Rightly or wrongly, I choose to save my energy. I tell her that in my opinion she is headed for trouble, affirm our availability, and ask her what she will do if things go wrong. Feeling newly redeemed, she has not yet imagined this possibility.

Throughout our dialogue the patient's bright, verbal five-year-old son has been the leitmotif. Probably "adultified" beyond his years by the life he has led, he has chimed in with articulate opinions about his mother's treatment, her friendships, her living situation—even while squirming in her lap. At first endearing, the boy's precocity becomes almost eerie over time. But sensing the downward trend in my conversation with his mother, I have tried to engage him now and again to keep a lighter feeling going and show my continued good will toward this family of two. "Can I color?" he asks, and I offer clinic stationery and a Depakote pen, telling him that I like to color, too. As the visit draws to a close, I look towards the boy.

"You're living for more than just yourself now," I say to the patient. "You are not being responsible as a parent to take your psychiatric treatment into your own hands." With a final patriarchal flourish I state that I will be considering whether to ask Child Protective to reopen the case (not that this would realistically accomplish anything).

I have now "acted out" and given the patient the scolding lecture she'd expected. I reiterate our continued availability and as she storms out I leave her with the words, "Take care of him."

But the boy does not leave. Even when I tell him he can take his "coloring" with him, he keeps working, glued to my desk till mother returns to retrieve him. I flatter myself that he is somehow voting for me and my genuine concern, my truth-telling. More likely this is just one more uncomfortable scene involving his mother, from which he adeptly dissociates.

And it's on to the next patient.

• • • • •

It has been a dry spring in Maine. Two weeks after writing the above, as overdue rain falls outside the same office window, I laugh at the irony of my opening homily on "saving energy," since clearly both my admonition to the patient, and the essay I started afterwards, have absorbed plenty. With the relief of the rain I can accept my scripted role as a foil for this young woman's anger. Her drive to develop was bound to extract energy from me one way or the other.

Irreducibly we are both trapped within the human condition. She has an illness and cannot trust; she will get help only in dire need. When relatively "well" she will want to resume her development as a self. With her history of constant invalidation by powerful adults, she has to do this by asserting her own independent worldview, even if this worldview derives from the Birkenstock-shod marketing machine of the multi-million dollar herbal medicine industry; even if it will lead her back into psychiatric illness. What she needs most is for me and all I represent to be wrong.

If she is trapped between her illness and the vicissitudes of development, I am trapped in the script of the Helper, simultaneously wanting to act, to save, and overwhelmed by the Savior's role. This familiar paradigm has a 2000-year precedent, though I can blame my lot on more immediate circumstances.

I can blame, for example, the "split therapy" structure of clinic work. The case manager and I are both good at what we do, but she, the case worker, represents support without authority, and I, the doctor, am authority without support. Wouldn't the patient stand a better chance of learning how to trust if these two functions were deftly combined?

Perhaps. But I have put in years with such patients doing just that in private practice, so I can't pretend that the effort wouldn't be even more overwhelming—or that it would necessarily work. With some patients, it has; with others, I've sometimes wondered what value the effort had aside from that of furthering my own education (much as Winnicott used to speak of doing "research analysis").

And anyway, this is the clinic. Here we can only hope that this patient's cycle of approach-in-sickness/avoidance-in-health attenuates before she is destroyed.

Whether this individual survives intact or not, the life force embodied in her development is inexorable. The leaves outside draw water into themselves, unfurling in the rain just as she drew my energy, against my will, into the necessary role. My actions, I see now, crystallized around my identification with her intellectually overdeveloped son, always trying to say and do the right thing to keep his mother functioning. His, finally, is the role I'm still in. Who takes care of us?

GOD OR VENDING MACHINE?

Dr. Peter Kramer was among the first to publicly observe that the Prozac family of new antidepressant/antipanic drugs (SSRIs) ushered our culture into a new era. A decade later, it is hard to remember how America functioned without them and their successors. Like nature's chemicals, these manmade ones are morally neutral, merely opening new possibilities for how humans experience, or construct, what is meaningful in their lives. There is no one right attitude to take toward their influence, only individual situations, like these cases, to ponder. It would be easier (but a lot less interesting) if the partisans for or against a simplistic "biological psychiatry" had a monopoly on the truth.

This piece appeared in the February 1998 *Psychiatric Times*.

Two middle-aged men; two cases of DSM-IV "Panic Disorder." Both respond beautifully to SSRIs as far as major symptoms go, but I finally come to such different judgments about each situation that I am led to wonder whether the prescribing psychiatrist's role is best conceived as that of God or of psychopharmacologic vending machine.

The first patient I have known for many years, some of which have been spent in intensive psychotherapy without maintenance medication. Panic and anticipatory anxiety typically involved group situations wherein this accomplished professional would present his ideas or advocate for his position. Sometimes his symptoms would force him to leave important meetings, or prevent him, marooned in roadside panic en route, from arriving. He is an "idea man": a creative introvert who happens to most enjoy thinking about certain problems which have important public policy implications. Since "public policy" today is largely made in the privacy of corporate boardrooms rather than the more observable context of legislatures and courts, my patient's expertise and intellectual passion places him in a perpetual dilemma.

His ideas draw him recurrently to participate, to be a "player" in a competitive corporate world for which he is temperamentally unsuited. Those most successful at accomplishing their agendas in this world (as my patient, plausibly, tells it) are motivated most by the pleasures of obtaining and exercising power and less concerned with the content of what they are trying to accomplish. They are extraverted, politically adept, and varying degrees of charming and ruthless. Someone like my patient, who lapses into thinking that actual ideas and their implications are the central issue, is repeatedly brought up short when he wakens to the power game he is inadvertently playing (and often losing). Far from thriving on it, he is overstressed and finally panicked by it.

Over the years, by way of an interesting and useful developmental inquiry, we have both satisfied ourselves that, while his history may have accentuated his tendency towards anxiety, a large part of his vulnerability is not negotiable. The panic which has come and gone from various periods of his life is part of "who he is," the symptomatic extension of a wary introverted nature which is either genetically founded and/or neurophysiologically embedded from pre-verbal or even prenatal experience. This conclusion leads naturally to the notion of constructing a life around this trait, thus adapting to it. And in fact the patient has done just that for a couple of long stretches, suffering only minimal symptoms unmedicated during those periods.

The adaptation has been that of a quasi-academic freelance consultant and writer, with home office, fax, and more lately, Web site: the sort of cottage industry, in fact, that many of us surviving psychotherapists currently engage in. In his field, however, this safe contemplative haven, while it offers a decent living, is not a position from which he can really influence the course of the large policy issues that are his passion. So like moth to flame he is drawn back to the corporate dominance hierarchy (dressed up though it may be in the garb of post-industrial "high-touch" teamwork) and gets burned again.

This last round, reluctantly, my patient returned in search of SSRI maintenance (one of them had been briefly successful before). He was also looking for a way to think about what all this meant and to decide whether to once again exit the corporate arena as quickly as possible, or not. It comes down to what he wants to do with his life. Clearly his field is truly his "calling" and he will feel unfulfilled without pursuing it. But it is equally clear that his temperament or "type" does not fit the contemporary interpersonal context within which that calling must be pursued. This confounded SSRI, itself the creature of a corporate laboratory, offers him an option to stay and to be effective. Should he take it?

Shrink-like, I could of course simply turn the question back to him. (Perhaps this "shrinking" from a personal response is another root of our profession's slang title.) Knowing that he wants to hear from me, I do not. I wish to conceal neither my values or the ways in which those values lead me to admire his honest concern for the public good. So I simply label my response as a personal rather than a "professional" one.

I reflect that, by artificial chemical means, the SSRI allows him to "live against type" and that in doing so he brings a different mentality and a different set of priorities to bear on an issue that affects us all; an attitude which I trust and which might help to balance the power-motivations of those who now make most of the decisions. (Peter Kramer has speculated somewhat optimistically that psychopharmacology could be a "politically progressive force" by allowing people like this patient to challenge the intrinsically dominant.)

In other cultures and times, I continue, creative introverts may have been afforded more societally influential roles, while having their contemplative lifestyles respected. Here I wonder about shamans in our ancestral hunter-gatherer bands or think of the great Sioux religious leader Black Elk, whose visions were incorporated into his group's decision-making.

Our society offers no such niche. If my patient wishes to influence important immediate events in his domain, he will need my help and the SSRI's help to do so. And if that is his choice I will support it with my expertise and prescribing authority. And a voice within me asks, "Since when do you get to play God?"

I tell myself that I am not making the decision for him, knowing full well that I have provided a frame for it that he would not have come up with on his own. My judgment is twofold: first, that he will be recurrently drawn to the flame anyway, and second, that it is better to state my own values explicitly rather than hide behind a fiction of objectivity. This last takes his high level of psychological functioning into account. I don't pretend that it is without transferential risks. In his case, I estimate the risks of "objectivity" to be greater.

The second patient was seen more briefly as a "med consult" favor to a psychologist friend. Also from the corporate sector, he was just the sort of politically savvy "player" that might intimidate the first. At home in the outer world of power, he developed panic attacks only upon being drawn into a less familiar, inner world of feeling by a younger male coworker who saw him and reached him as no one had before. In late middle age, this patient was at the top of his field, many years married and socially well known; he felt able neither to abandon himself to this new kind of intimacy nor to renounce it. He was good at secrets but not at intense inner conflict, and wasn't sure how much more he could risk jeopardizing his outward life by discovering more about his potential for openness, contact, and new dimensions of sexual identity.

All of this found a common pathway through his locus ceruleus; he sought medication to buy himself some time, to slow things down. Once again an SSRI did the trick. But as the months wore on and he no longer had symptoms severe enough to move him in any direction, he seemed to settle into his double life more or less indefinitely. Since all he wanted was maintenance, I turned him over to his family physician on the ready rationale that I generally don't follow people for meds alone. The deeper truth was that I was uncomfortable supporting what seemed at the time like a non-resolution of his psychological problem. But this emotional reaction to his "duplicity" derived, once again, from my own (this time, unexamined) values and not from an objective source. From a retrospective and value-neutral perspective his was no less a resolution than the first patient's. His choice was simply to live, for better or worse, through chemistry, adapting via one available option. My personal values led me to support the first patient's decision to transcend his intrinsic biological capacity to contain a dilemma, but not the second patient's. I did not moralize to the latter but bowed out and have lost touch since. I suppose that playing God is more appealing than playing vending machine.

REQUIEM FOR
PSYCHOANALYSIS

**Alan Stone (introduced below) is a brilliant and scrupulous elder states-
man of psychiatry and psychoanalysis; one with whose opinions I
strongly differed here. I include this topical piece (published as "Alan
Stone's Requiem for Psychoanalysis" in the May 1997 *Psychiatric
Times*) less for the debate with Stone than for its capsule description
of, and advocacy for, what I consider to be the essence of psychoanalytic psychotherapy.**

From the cover of this winter's issue of *Harvard Magazine,* that most reproduced and caricatured of twentieth century visages—Freud's bearded face—
peers forth. "Psychoanalysis failed as science. Will it survive as art?" asks the
caption. But the featured article isn't just one more popularized rehash of
familiar scandals. The author of this serious essay (originally an address to the
American Academy of Psychoanalysis) is Alan Stone, M.D.: Harvard professor,
Boston Institute graduate, former president of the American Psychiatric
Association. In it, after establishing that analysis is "an interpretive discipline
rather than a natural science," Stone goes on to make a damning statement
about analysis as medical treatment. First, since the major DSM axis I syndromes cannot be linked to specific disruptions of psychoanalytic developmental stages, there is "no reason to assume that a careful reconstruction of
those ... events will have a therapeutic effect." And if patients' memories of the
past cannot be trusted to be literally true (as the sex-abuse hysteria of the last
decade made clear), then therapy should focus "almost entirely on the here and
now, on problem-solving." Psychoanalysis, says Stone, will survive not as a
treatment for psychiatric and medical symptoms—for which it is inadequate—
but as an elective means of exploring the self and dealing with "ordinary
human suffering." That last is a pointed reversal of Freud's original statement:
that ordinary suffering would be what was left after successful treatment.

In short, Stone, in an influential forum, chooses to contribute his own shove to the de-coupling of psychoanalysis from psychiatric medicine.

Why should I care? I have never trusted institutionalized psychoanalysis; never accepted the supposed legitimacy conferred by that deadening look-alike row of Freud's *Collected Works* on the analyst's bookshelf, nor assumed the supposed sanity conferred by his framed institute certificate. I still recall Freud's Viennese friend and trainee, Richard Sterba, telling my residency class that with his independence of mind, Freud would have been unlikely to survive a contemporary analytic institute. Of my own two personal therapies, the one not conducted by a formally credentialed analyst went at least as deep and, for me, was equally worthy of the term "analysis."

In many ways it is easier to survey the damage analysis has done to psychiatry than to defend it. Psychoanalyst/historian Philip Cushman gives a convincing account of its rise in this country, springboarding from the earlier, homegrown "mental hygiene" movement. As consumer capitalism increasingly permeated the American psyche, psychoanalysis unwittingly ensured that the psyche's ills would remain private (not social and political) concerns and that a purchasable commodity—itself—would be available to address them. Thus, though derived from a somewhat disreputable movement founded by a European Jew, the American analysts of the 1950s arrived at the ideological center of this country's power structure, bearing the legitimizing stamp of medical science. (It was they and not Freud himself who insisted that analysts must be physicians.)

So it is small wonder that a psychoanalyst like Alan Stone, trained during that heyday, would mourn the loss of conviction that made his teacher, John Murray, compare his own refinements in psychoanalytic theory to the placing of one brick in "Freud's cathedral." Such disillusionment resembles that of Skid Row ballads from the Great Depression: "Once I lived the life of a millionaire...." But in dismissing the practical therapeutic value of all that quaint stuff about dreams and transference and development, Stone is throwing the baby out with the bath water.

Let the bath water go. If analysis is worth anything, it is as a means of helping people, not as a beautiful cultural artifact like the cathedral at Chartres. The dogmatic inflexibility of much analytic theory is more aptly compared to another medieval religious phenomenon, Scholasticism, whose monks spent five centuries doing such things as classifying animal species from normative ideal categories in lieu of walking through the woods observing them. Until the last couple of decades, analysis succeeded in keeping the rest of psychology out of psychiatry, marginalizing theories and treatments that did not conform instead of attempting to seriously engage them. Thus, psychoanalysis as an institution dug its own grave, preparing the way for the current biochemical ascendancy and its mechanical psychotherapeutic imitators.

The problem is not that analysis is an "interpretive discipline" rather than a natural science as currently defined. Instead, the problem is that institutionalized psychoanalysis is a *rigid* interpretive discipline that has not evolved to maintain its usefulness or yield to observed facts.

Thus, the whole idea of an interpretive discipline within psychiatry and medicine has been discredited just when (as biological psychiatry reaches inevitable limits) we need it the most. Today's psychiatric trainees are deprived of an important tool and a unique joy: the ability to think interpretively about their patients. With this level of abstraction absent they are either reduced to psychopharmacological tinkering alone, or forced to import New Age truisms from the popular culture. Is it any surprise that their numbers are shrinking!

I do not make the argument for interpretation on academic grounds, which I believe are misleading. I make it on the grounds of clinical usefulness.

Freud, both a genius and a flawed man with gaping holes in his self-awareness, left us not just with his theory but with a method. Talk to patients over time, he said, and the relationship you form will offer clues about unconscious, habitual patterns of cognition and feeling that the patients carry with them. Try and trace these patterns back to their origin, "there and then," in developmental history. And listen to dreams—they are the Royal Road to understanding.

Over and over again, in a typically once-a-week context I am not permitted to call analysis, I have seen these simple but radical principles deliver definitive help. They have, at times, cured axis I syndromes. Even when they have not they have often released patients into more fulfilling and effective lives and relationships.

No, the method is not universally successful, and it has its risks. In this it favorably compares to other medical treatments. No, it does not cure schizophrenia, nor is there the simple one-to-one correspondence between developmental "fixations" and adult illness that the 1950s cathedral-builders fantasized. But, as analyst/infant researcher Daniel Stern's work shows, the history of the child's developing self is critically relevant to the individualized treatment of axis I disorders, regardless of diagnosis. No, this method is no substitute for the appropriate use of medications. But I have seen it succeed in cases of, for example, mysteriously recurrent "refractory depression" where one-dimensional biological treatment could not.

A European psychiatrist once observed that, as war is too important to be left to the generals, psychoanalysis too important to be left to the psychoanalysts. It is time to reclaim the essential elements of the method for psychiatry itself. What of Stone's question about memory? If we are academics, either memory is "true" like experimental results, or it is "constructed" as narrative text. Since the first alternative is obviously an oversimplification, Stone concludes that analysis is a literary activity, bolstering his argument with the fact that psychoanalytic theory today is most often taught in humanities courses rather than medical school. So, if not to the analysts, should we leave analysis to the literary critics?

Only if we are academics. As pragmatic clinicians we need not succumb to such a false polarity. The act of memory can often give us a plausible account, perhaps not of literal facts from early childhood but of recurrent patterns within a family and their emotional impact on the patient. To say that such an account is entirely a "constructed" product of the clinical dyad is to equate (for example) incest-memory adventurism with responsible exploratory psychotherapy. I believe there is a difference and that I can effectively guard (and warn patients to guard) against injecting too much of my own constructions into my patients' histories.

If I do not make such an effort to investigate "there and then" or if I restrict myself to Stone's practical problem-solving in the here-and-now, I often fall into a trap and become part of a pathological system. If I accept a patient's conscious perceptions and goals (as opposed to her pain) at face value, I may be ignoring her most fundamental problem. Karen Horney—who, like many of our most creative analysts, was cast out of the orthodox establishment—characterized it thus: "Patients come not to rid themselves of their neuroses, but to *perfect* them." I cannot believe that psychoanalyst Alan Stone has forgotten this principle or that his own work is really as simple-minded as his article makes it sound.

The Richard Dreyfuss character in the movie farce *What About Bob?* perfectly personifies all that needs to die in psychoanalysis. He combines in one character the slavish worship of Freud (bust on the mantle, clipped beard) with the fatuous pop-psychology to which analysis has ghettoized the rest of psychotherapy. His "exemplary" adjustment is laughably contrived. Let it die; down the drain, I say.

The real work is to clarify, salvage, and demystify all that is true and even noble about the past century's encounter with the Unconscious. Fortunately, this necessary effort is already underway, though not yet coherently organized with a common vocabulary. Using the efficient and clinically flexible tool of deliberately metaphorical thinking, several writers are building interpretive models capable of generating clinical hypotheses and predictions that can be confirmed or disconfirmed without worrying overmuch about whether or not they are doing "science." I see a remarkable convergence, for example, between the work of James Gustafson, who has distilled his theory from the analytic tradition, and that of Marcia Linehan, a "cognitive-behaviorist" who in essence has reinvented psychodynamics from scratch. Like these authors, even the cryptic analyst Michael Eigen seems to be focusing lately on "the thing that does not change" (Eigen's words).

Instead of holding out the promise of conflicts that can be resolved and done with or deficits that can be replaced by "re-parenting," this emerging interpretive paradigm sees human problems as "dialectical dilemmas" (Linehan) that can only be more and more consciously inhabited. The lesson of a hundred years of analysis seems to be that there are some ways in which people can change and some in which they will not. Interpretation, as much as biochemical manipulation and good advice, will remain a potent means of changing the things that can be changed and adapting to those that cannot.

THE SHIFTING METAPHORS
OF BIOLOGICAL PSYCHIATRY

It is easy to dismiss the real progress biological psychiatry has made based on the oversimplistic way that it is typically used. Some therapists loudly do so and then make their "medication referrals" more quietly. Here I look at both sides of the equation with purposely opposite clinical vignettes.

The "diagnosis *du jour,*" be it Multiple Personality in the 1980s, Attention Deficit Hyperactivity Disorder in the 1990s, or whatever comes next, tends to reflect global socioeconomic themes and is therefore invariably overapplied. Unwitting agents of history, some of the Authorities of the day build their careers on it... until the next cultural shift. Those who stay in the game long enough learn that diagnoses are often secondary when it comes to understanding and helping individuals.

"Metaphors" appeared in the September 1996 *Psychiatric Times.*

The patient, a successful thirty-five-year-old educator, is seeking my expert opinion. This will be her third psychiatric rendering, and I am going to disappoint her. Psychiatrist #1 diagnosed her with "adult Attention-Deficit Hyperactivity Disorder" and tried her on stimulants and antidepressants (this is a patient who earlier obtained her Ph.D. from a rigorous program in just two and a half years). Psychiatrist #2 thought her to be a "rapid-cycling bipolar" and so now as she speaks she carries a therapeutic level of valproic acid [trade name Depakote, today's standard mood stabilizer]. Neither intervention has been definitively successful; which doctor is right? I feel as if I am supposed to deliver the tie-breaking diagnosis from behind door number three.

The setup may be amusing, but the patient's suffering is real. An intelligent and ambitious woman, she is hamstrung between competing visions of a fulfilling life, trying to juggle small children, a demanding job, and a husband who wants to have a relationship with her. She's been dropping the ball

114

lately—snapping angrily at people at home and on the job, sleeping poorly, drinking too much coffee in the morning and wine at night.

Psychiatrists have not been her only recourse. She's read books about how to relax and how to prioritize. Maybe, she decided, a career change would help. So when a well-liked local restaurant went on the market, she took a serious look. For a period of weeks she stayed up as late as midnight, after her husband had turned in, pouring over the eatery's financial records. After an accountant friend gave her some free advice, she abandoned the idea of becoming a restaurateur and became dejected and unenthusiastic around the house again.

Psychiatrist #2 had seen this restaurant episode and her previous, more sustained high-energy period in graduate school, as hypomanic episodes followed by periods of depression. I could follow his reasoning and certainly couldn't say for certain that he was wrong. What was more clear to me was that each project—first graduate school and later, the restaurant—was a product of desperation, an attempt to find a purpose for what often felt like an empty and meaningless life. And each led to a crushing deflation when its "solution" failed. Sources for such feelings were hinted at in her developmental and substance abuse histories. Of course psychiatrist #2 could easily conjecture that these very histories were themselves the products of an underlying biologically based mood instability.

Where psychiatrist #1 had come up with ADHD in such an accomplished individual, I couldn't honestly fathom (I am told that "hyperfocus" is a new permutation on this ever-widening diagnosis). But it interested me that stimulants, whose effects I would expect to support the patient's conscious intention to continue in "fast-forward," didn't seem to satisfy her. She'd become even more irritable, more acutely sensitive to perceived demands. Had simply adding energy to a conflicted psyche backfired?

This case typifies my psychiatric practice here at century's end. When I began in the early 1980s, occasional patients were still coming in diagnosing themselves with an oedipus complex. Today they often arrive equipped with a biological disease, sometimes even bearing the results of standardized symptom questionnaires. The problem here is not that these shifting diagnoses may be incomplete or wrong. It is that they close off further inquiry into our patients' lives, substituting scientific literalism for story and encouraging them to accept someone else's label in lieu of understanding themselves in their own terms.

In supplying the above patient with a ready-made diagnosis—be it ADHD or rapid-cycling bipolar disorder—we are handing her a metaphor. A disease of inadequate focus or of roller-coaster moods "explains" the situation she finds herself in. The larger neurochemical metaphor—"you are a broken machine"—leads us away from considerations of meaning, i.e., What was getting a Ph.D. supposed to do for her? What would it mean to own a restaurant? Her strivings have become only symptoms. Aside from availing herself of a psychopharmacologist, she is disempowered from affecting these symptoms.

It is not as if we have a choice about using metaphors: They are our fundamental mode of comprehending complex phenomena. Contemporary physicists who discuss the "color" of subatomic particles know this as surely as postmodern psychoanalysts. Newtonian physics is taken literally not because it is "real" but because it is an extremely accurate and useful metaphor under everyday observed conditions. Likewise deficit theories of depression or ADHD (as research neurochemists know). If a car is coming at me, I will clearly act according to the classical Newtonian metaphor to avoid being killed. If someone is suicidal and melancholic, I will prescribe antidepressants. But when the above patient presents, it seems far less clear what the most helpful metaphor will be.

I tell the patient I will need more time and a therapeutic relationship of some sort with her in order to comfortably offer an opinion on how best to approach her problem. I certainly do not rule out the potential usefulness of medication but want to be skeptical about any labeling such use might imply and, if possible, to hold off for awhile on new prescriptions in order to better understand her situation as it stands. Time will tell whether I am only imagining a deeper relief beneath her initial frustration. She does schedule with me again.

It would be easy to end this essay here. Yet for the sake of honesty, I feel obligated to present an opposite case to illustrate just how puzzling it can be to sail in the shifting winds of present-day psychiatry.

The patient is a forty-year-old alternative medical practitioner who has already had extensive Jungian-oriented therapy. Medications and medical-psychiatric labels are the furthest thing from his mind; he is here for additional long-term analytic work with no expectation of "cure." Yet as I get to know him over many months I am struck by how much a slave to Meaning (capital "M") he is. When he descends into forty-eight or seventy-two-hour hells of lifelessness, helpless sobbing, wishing he were dead, he searches compulsively for the core psychological/spiritual issue—the "something" that is "up." Resourceful as he is, he can usually discover something new about himself, and I join him in his efforts, for which he is grateful. Such is our therapeutic contract. Conversely, when he emerges with a burst of creative energy and physical vitality, he often seems to credit his new insight for the reprieve, as if he had finally gotten to the rightest, deepest stuff. And this sets himself up for disappointment when the next descent catches him unawares.

This patient's lifestyle and profession afford him the flexibility to tolerate such moodswings without chemical modification, and I have no investment in prescribing valproate for him or giving him a "rapid-cycler" diagnosis. In fact, for a long time I avoid explicit mention of these last for fear of alienating him (eventually I offer them, for the sake of completeness). It is clear he values the intensity of his experiences both positive and negative; that these threaten no-one; and that he enjoys being who he is most of the time. But my inner biological psychiatrist has not gone to sleep. In this patient's case I am feeling that the quest for Meaning may itself be damaging, diverting his valuable energy into self-blame and existential dread when he is down and giving him a false sense of security when he is up. I don't need to worry about this man's abandoning his lifelong effort to understand himself. A biological metaphor is called for.

Consider the possibility, I suggest, that these awful lows and energetic highs don't always have to *mean* something. What if, like the nature outside you, the nature inside your skin is subject to a kind of "weather." Weather changes when it will, and we can sacrifice a goat in hopes of influencing it, or we can give up controlling and learn to anticipate it and to build shelters and wear clothes to help ourselves withstand it. (This latter is the category that mood-stabilizing medication would fall into, if such became necessary.) We learn a lot from existing in the weather—our inner landscape can appear very differently in storm, fog, snow, sun—but the weather will always be there as an Other beyond our power.

As I see it, this patient had been enculturated into a worldview that understanding equals control. His desperate desire to "understand" in this way made eminent sense given the severity of his mood variations. Yet paradoxically, as he absorbs my biological (but not mechanical) metaphor, his cycles seem to be receding in significance. When he is down he concentrates more on just getting through it; when up, more on building a solid life for fair weather and foul.

Have I encouraged this patient to close off inquiry into meaning—the very move I criticized in my account of the first patient's diagnostic adventures? I don't think so. I think he is finding a humbler, small "m" meaning in his new awareness of a reality external to his ego which is non-negotiable. This is the very same reality of which our own medical doctors so often need to remind us.

I don't know whether I can convincingly reconcile the seeming contradiction in my work with these two patients who had been enculturated into such different languages within our mental health Tower of Babel. In this business, one does what works and intellectualizes after the fact. After the fact, the common themes I find are these: 1) my conscious awareness of the inevitable use of metaphor in both cases, 2) a desire not to close off inquiries into meaning too soon, and 3) a specific desire to avoid an overly mechanical version of the biological metaphor. Machines are made by men and women; weather and women and men are made by Nature.

If we try to banish metaphors, they will go underground and influence us unconsciously. But a recognition of the inevitability of metaphor makes our work more effective. A neuroscience which honored metaphor might even take some cues from our clinical work. I think here of how many colleagues I know who use variations of the metaphor of "steerage" to explain to their patients the subjective phenomena of depression. "It's like trying to paddle a half-swamped canoe." "Like sailing upwind without a keel." "Like trying to drive a truck without power steering." "Like trying to turn a bicycle when you haven't got up enough speed." We are easily overwhelmed, thrown off course, and exhaust ourselves in the attempt to get back on track.

Surely these time-tested metaphors say something accurate about the biochemical derangements in those neurotransmitter systems which regulate the background reactive tone of neural networks. If the neuroscientists would ask us clinicians more about how we work with patients, they would doubtless find some specific inspiration for their research.

The trade in biological metaphors could stand to be a more two-way street.

THE COMING POLARIZATION
OF PSYCHOTHERAPY

"As the therapy culture splits, the richer metaphors of growth and relational healing will rarely be available outside a discrete market niche, while those without gold cards will find only store-brand messages of conformity, work functioning, and symptom suppression." Viewed from where I now write, what I foresaw in the May 1995 *Psychiatric Times* has largely come to pass. (Of course, now the cards are platinum.) And yet, a surprising number of therapists continue to work and think independently, outside of these polarities, keeping faith with their patients.

I include the piece primarily for its two cases: Tolstoy's, and that of his modern counterpart.

In the first days of September, 1869, Count Leo Nikolayevich Tolstoy, armed with the early royalties from his *War and Peace*, journeyed several hundred miles from his ancestral estate to buy additional lands. This trip was his latest effort at that most ancient of coping strategies: distraction. He was forty-one, and his fear of death had been rapidly intensifying in recent months. "It came on him all of a sudden—he began to tremble, sweat broke out on his forehead, he felt a presence behind his back." On the final carriage ride, the Russian countryside itself seemed to turn hostile, and when he could go no further he took a room at an inn in a village called Arzamas. While his servant slept in the hallway, the room became for Tolstoy a "square red and white tomb."

> "This is ridiculous," I told myself. "Why am I so depressed? What am I afraid of?"
>
> "Of me," answered Death. "I am here." A cold shudder ran over my skin. Yes, Death. It will come, it is already here, even though it has nothing to do with me now ... My whole

being ached with the need to live, the right to live, and, at the same moment, I felt death at work. And it was awful being torn apart inside. I tried to shake off my terror. I found the stump of a candle in a brass candlestick and lighted it. The reddish flame, the candle, the candlestick, all told me the same story: there is nothing in life, nothing in life, nothing exists but death, and death should not be! [quoted in introduction to *Ilyich*, p. 25]

The Count's death anxieties, of which this episode was one recorded climax, were to dominate him for years to come. He finally emerged from them—after a nine-year period during which he was unable to write fiction following the publication of *Anna Karenina*—at age fifty-seven, with the terse novella *The Death of Ivan Illyich*. *Illyich* is a classic example of what the English psychoanalyst Elliot Jacques called "sculpted creativity" in his pioneering essay, "Death and the Mid-Life Crisis." From this point, Tolstoy's literary powers were restored and the extreme death-fears receded. Tolstoy portrayed a character who, in his final moments, discovers that love, "the real thing," is greater than death. Illyich finds this love in his son's touch.

Tolstoy's example will serve us as a reference point presently.

Carl Jung's description of polarities holds true whether we are discussing a problem experienced by a particular patient in psychotherapy or, as here, a problem that now confronts the field of psychotherapy itself:

> "...[A]ll the greatest and most important problems of life are fundamentally insoluble. They must be so, for they express the necessary polarity inherent in every self-regulating system. They can never be solved, but only outgrown."

History, technological advances, and market economics are now forcing our field into a set of false polarities (see table). These two conflicting orientations, each of which *seems* coherent and internally consistent, distract us from our primary loyalty: the health of our patients. If we fail to become aware of these polarities inhabiting our profession, we will be split by them into two less effective halves. As individual practitioners our best chance for surviving the coming confusion will be to find our own unique ways of defining our work outside the tyranny of either preconceived orientation. We will take up the perils of each in turn.

The idea that mental symptoms are meaningless afflictions, obstacles to the ego's worldly agenda which treatment should quickly remove or suppress, has gained credibility with the ascendancy of psychopharmacology, brief focused therapies, and managed mental health care. Some therapeutic implications of this conception are represented on the right-hand side of the table.

120

The False Polarities
(limiting preconceptions about psychotherapy held by therapists and/or patients)

Symptoms
are valuable and meaningful (but what if they can't be withstood?)

Symptoms
are meaningless impediments (but what if they don't go away?)

The Process
is one of soul-searching: a narrative dialogue through which both people change

The Process
is one of focused problem-solving: doctor "fixes" patient by the application of diagnosis-specific technique(s)

The Starting Point
"not knowing": curiosity, open-ended exploration

The Starting Point
formulation of the problem: (biological, psychodynamic, systemic, etc.)

The Duration
long-term; potentially, a way of life

The Duration
time-limited

The Ideal Outcome
is character change, restoration of the Self

The Ideal Outcome
is symptom relief as a measurable goal

Individuation
is a unique differentiation against the backdrop of a universal human condition

Good Adjustment
is an adaptive niche within contemporary culture, judged by social and workplace effectiveness

Therapists
are personally initiated into the ways of the psyche: wisdom

Therapists
are technically trained and credentialed: knowledge

The Therapy Subculture
claims to subvert prevailing social norms, but most available to the socioeconomically privileged

Behavioral Health Care
is part of the medical/psychological mainstream and the healthcare industry: wider availability

The Faithful Person
trusts that life will lead him/her

The Self-Confident Person
makes informed choices to lead a better life

Let us pluck Tolstoy from the Russian steppe and bring him to a modern academic medical center. The clinical interview and rating scales classify his terror as DSM-IV Panic Disorder. A cognitive therapist tries to "de-catastrophize" his maladaptive thought patterns. Desipramine or sertraline dampens his state of overarousal and stems his obsessively morbid ruminations. [These antidepressants are among the standard treatments for panic attacks.] His wife, who in her own journals bluntly wrote of her husband's "disease," is pleased to find the Count restored to her as an emotionally available partner, rather than the eccentric would-be saint he eventually became.

But whether epiphanies like the night at Arzamas would have occurred, whether *Ivan Illyich* would have been written—whether Tolstoy would have finally transcended his fear of death—none of us can say.

As the symptomatic relief of mental anguish becomes ever more refined, suffering is demoted from destiny to inconvenience. The notion that pain shapes the soul sounds antiquated; one might say it is a defensive religious rationalization from the pre-antidepressant era. Few people believe anymore that symptoms can have a symbolic meaning; fewer still, a transformative purpose.

We find Peter Kramer, in the latter pages of *Listening to Prozac*, attesting to the virtues of "hyperthymic creativity" as opposed to the dysthymic variety. Yet just as Kramer is unable to convincingly shake his dour foil, the Catholic writer Walker Percy, many of us are unable to forget that a preponderance of the greatest works of art and most profound insights into the human condition have their origins in desperation.

I spoke several years ago with Martin Seligman, originator of the famous "learned helplessness" experiments, at a conference where he was presenting on the cognitive therapy of depression. "None of this has anything to do with wisdom," he said of these techniques which are so frequently effective in improving mental and physical health. "The depressed organism is probably the more accurate transducer of reality."

Whatever healing Tolstoy may have achieved was won without sacrificing such accuracy. His protracted struggle with death might be called a "healing crisis," a term borrowed from classical acupuncture. Winnicott's essay "Fear of Breakdown" expresses its nature in our more familiar, developmental metaphor.

Winnicott would say that Tolstoy's panics—"primitive agonies" was the analyst's preferred name for them—brought "a past situation into the present tense" so that it could be experienced for the first time by a developed self. This situation was the annihilation, or psychic death, which the inadequately buffered or traumatized infant experiences psychosomatically (Tolstoy's mother died when he was twenty-three months old; he was raised by a succession of relatives thereafter). The developed, verbal self is better equipped to metabolize the perception of raw, unmediated reality which overwhelmed and fragmented its infant predecessor. Psychotherapy is one transitional space within which this can occur; artistic creation is another.

Tolstoy did not overcome his fear of death by psychological means—acquiring more positive cognitions, the illusion of a safer and fairer world. Nor was it overcome by an exogenous alteration in his neurotransmitter balance (though such alteration may have resulted, endogenously). Tolstoy's was a spiritual healing in that it recognized and deferred to the incomprehensible power of a universe in which his ego's agenda was without final significance. Tolstoy learned that he was not leading his life, but rather, his life was leading him. This accomplished, he had less need to be led by symptoms.

Few of us have the inner strength and creative intelligence that Tolstoy needed to survive in this way, without pills, therapists, or credible priests. Vodka and an early grave was the more likely outcome among his contemporaries; the Count himself remained a distorted and at times, destructive personality. Yet the lessons that the Tolstoys, the William Blakes, the Abraham Lincolns—and the neighborhood survivor/sages—give us are as alien hieroglyphics to those who see human mental anguish only as a meaningless impediment. Will a society led by well-adapted, illusion-prone optimists rather than Abraham Lincolns cope as well with unforeseen challenges?

Reacting to the shallowness of mechanistic approaches, many thoughtful patients, wanting to understand their symptoms, abandon the medical mainstream. The alternatives available to these seekers after meaning are suggested by the left-hand half of the table. Were he alive today, Tolstoy would likely have been among these people (assuming he could overcome his distaste for doctors of all sorts, whom he called "clerks"). His introspectiveness would be necessary but not sufficient for him to make this choice; the options referred to generically as "depth psychotherapy" depend increasingly upon patients' secure financial status. As our therapy culture splits, the richer metaphors of growth and relational healing will rarely be available outside a discrete market niche, while those without gold cards will find only store-brand messages of conformity, work functioning, and symptom suppression.

But let us bring the agonized Count to some representatives of the school of Meaning who work with the premises on the left of the table. Within psychiatry, one might pick a dissociationist; in the alternative world, that contemporary cultural icon, the Jungian analyst. If Tolstoy were able to ally with such therapists, his need to understand would be met by an interested other; his existential loneliness assuaged. A prolonged therapy might allow for the shaping of his soul in a more autonomous and individualized way, perhaps without the use of psychotropic drugs (or more likely, less use—in the mid-1990s even Jungians make "med referrals").

I wonder, though, whether the spare, direct imagery of *Ivan Illyich* would be diluted by more generic, "collective" imagery from world mythology or from the newer mythology of personality fragmentation. *Mysterium conjunctionis* or the fusion of part-selves? Either has a potential for being subtly orchestrated. The radically clear Russian vision of *Illyich* might be lost.

And again, what if, like most of us, Tolstoy had not been so strong? Despair, experienced from the inside, is a real and fundamental perception of the isolated ego which is so limited and battered. Symptoms may scream so loudly that no meaning can be made from them. The processes observed by depth psychologists and theologians offer no guarantees for the survival of the individual patient. From inside despair, an insistence on Journey and Process can at times ring sickeningly hollow, while honest attempts to relieve symptomatic suffering acquire more dignity.

At such junctures it may become necessary to adopt a stance of "knowing" and even of control—to use whatever techniques, drugs, and sometimes, credentialed authority we have at our disposal. The well-trained *and* initiated psychiatrist learns that compassion involves the responsible use of power as much as the avoidance of its misuse.

> "My heart starts to pound, my hands sweat. I close my eyes
> to calm myself, but all I feel is a void. My existence seems
> random and pointless and I feel like screaming."

The words of an American man at midlife with new-onset panic attacks recall Tolstoy. I have worked with this well-educated professional for several months. His symptoms have escalated to the point of jeopardizing his career, but up to now his reluctance to take medication has limited him to the occasional dose of benzodiazepine at his most desperate moments. He seeks to know why this is happening to him, and this search has led to insights into a life based upon pleasing others and its developmental origins. Nonetheless, this life he has made contains authentic elements: a solid marriage and loving, if somewhat distant, relationships with his children; socially valuable and rewarding work. He has had the impulse to throw it all away and go, alone, to the simpler context of a hunting camp or an *ashram*. But at the brink of losing everything he opts instead for a trial of an anti-panic medication, resolved that some of what he has is worth trying to save, by hook or by crook.

As the symptoms come under control, the void beneath them persists. In the following months, guided by his discoveries in therapy, he makes major external changes in his personal life and work routine without any sense that he is truly healing or understanding anything.

Then after a hiatus in the country he returns to describe a shift he noticed while looking at a tree: "It became so real and alive! Light and shadow on the bark, the ants crawling on it. When the leaves moved in the wind, I saw it as a being like myself." (How like Martin Buber in *I and Thou:* "[I]f will and grace are joined...as I contemplate the tree I am drawn into a relation, and the tree ceases to be an It.")

At irregular intervals other such experiences follow and begin to extend to people: children, wife, friends. He becomes less concerned with past and future and a kind of faith in his existence (but with no promise of a happy ending) creeps in. His panic symptoms subside. In another year he is off medication.

This patient's tree was not a symbol for something else. He saw it in its full, unmediated treeness. This led the way to an experience of self and other as real. I believe that any number of psychiatrists of varying orientations— the psychopharmacologist, the cognitive therapist, the self psychologist— might, in their own ways, have helped this patient into his new life. But *only* if they had been willing to suspend their theories, techniques and timetables and listen to him: first in his quest for meaning, then in his cry for symptom relief, and finally in his flickering vision of the living world.

I like to tell supervisees that therapy doesn't change people. Events change people. The task of therapy is to buffer events and turn them to the best possible use. Here I include symptoms as events: inner nature can be as uncontrollable and unknowable as outer nature can, despite the efforts of depth psychologists, biological psychiatrists, and purveyors of other theories and methods on either side of the table. Survival without shame, flesh-and-blood human connectedness—meanings with a small "m"—are more reliable guides for patient and therapist than either Meaning or Meaninglessness.

If we can cultivate a relationship that helps our patients (in Jung's phrase) "hang on until Nature grants a reprieve," then they stand the best chance of getting whatever message *may* be there for them in the screaming of the symptoms, in their own way, without being annihilated by it. Psychiatrists who stay true to the pragmatic traditions of their trade and do not allow themselves to be forced into a polarized outlook—who can move flexibly among several, variously useful points of view—are in a unique position to offer such help. Bleak as psychiatry's immediate future may seem, this presents us with a compelling opportunity.

P S Y C H I A T R I C   W I S D O M

The difference between knowledge and wisdom is always worth remembering. This piece was published as "What Is Psychiatric Wisdom?" in the August 1994 *Psychiatric Times*. It followed up on my debut article there a year before, which had struck a chord in our embattled profession, generating letters from demoralized psychiatrists around the country.

Eight years later it remains unclear whether the kind of psychiatry I speak for here will survive after my cohort of generalists are gone. However, we have learned a lot, and the patients we serve will always be here. I tried to capture the unique aspects of a pragmatic, medical ly based therapeutic discipline whose greatest strengths have been that of longitudinal naturalistic observation and a commitment to the relief of symptoms.

A year ago in these pages I published a rather gloomy article surveying the threats to our profession—external and internal to it—which have made the independently practicing psychiatrist an endangered species ["Is American Psychiatry Terminally Ill?" June 1993, opens Part IV below]. Today the situation has worsened to the point where I can no longer permit myself the luxury of pessimism. Some positive statement about psychiatry is called for, now. Those of us who are in mid-career will not be able to wait until we are fully ripened senior psychiatrists. As others concede defeat and predict the end of an era, we have been left to speak for and to define ourselves.

Is there any identity to this profession that still exists independent of our disparate fields of knowledge? Otherwise, why not have non-medical therapists do all the psychotherapy, family doctors and (soon) psychologists do the prescribing, neuroscience Ph.D.s do the brain research, and ethicists or theologians do the philosophizing? Why do some of us persist in loving this work as we have traditionally practiced it?

Is there such a thing as a wisdom that is specifically psychiatric?

Knowledge is what we build upon. In any field it is that sum to which we add new information and refined heuristic theories. Wisdom, by contrast, is timeless but easily forgotten. It is the truth of which we must always be reminded which is ignored and then rediscovered cyclically by succeeding generations. In its essence, wisdom is a subjectively validated inner experience rather than a set of transmissible data. Yet there is something that can be passed down: the places and situations wherein we have acquired it.

If we can find our way to a specifically psychiatric wisdom we will have arrived at a positive statement about our identity. And if not, we can at least point the way towards the lessons that will need to be relearned by the other health professionals destined to inherit the parceled-out fragments of our work. So I offer here my own unripened thoughts, drawing also on the experience of the many fine psychiatrists—students, teachers, peers—that I have known. For argument's sake I will begin with two important examples of what psychiatric wisdom is not.

Our wisdom is not psychopharmacology. While few would argue that pills can be complete practical solutions to human problems, we often tend to reason backwards from their effects to a simplistic (if unofficial) theory of mind, one which some of us still invoke with the words "chemical imbalance." At its worst, psychopharmacology as worldview gives us license to ignore the psychological and the spiritual. Materialist (so-called "biological") reductionism removes the search for story in our patient's lives. In its quest for control it misses the vital message, the meaning that may be transduced by symptoms.

But *wise* psychopharmacologists are willing to deal in a concrete and messy material world which many therapists would rather avoid. While their tools for the deciphering of meaning may be rudimentary, they do stand ready to join the battle against the destruction of lives by meaningless suffering. They admit the possibility of broken-ness and of irresolvable problems against which most psychological theories of health can be used as defense mechanisms.

Wise psychopharmacologists (I think of Hagop Akiskal quoting the blues lyrics of Memphis Slim) model for us the honor in palliation, the simple relief of suffering. They accept the sufferer as is, and in so doing avoid the pitfalls of another kind of reductionism: the idea that therapy done right can cure everything. They have learned to work patiently amid the shame and stigma surrounding "meds," ever aware of the biological vulnerabilities that in a moment can be revealed in any of us.

Recent scandals only confirm what cartoonists have always known: Wisdom is not inherent to psychoanalysis. Training in analytic institutes, however lengthy, costly, and inaccessible, confers neither ultimate authority, nor sanity, nor effectiveness upon its initiates. Instead, it may confer dangerous illusions of such attributes.

The analytic stance—whether closest to that of blank screen, trenchant interpreter, or empathic nurturer—reveals a fundamental ambivalence toward personal contact and power. Far from keeping the specifics of the analyst's self in a semi-opaque background, the very taking up of the analyst role speaks volumes about the analyst's personality and needs.

But, *wise* psychoanalysts are able to transcend these roles and make real contact without preconceptions. They help free the meaning contained in dreams and symptoms and restore (re-story) the narrative form to their patients' lives. Through their long collaboration with patients they have gained an immense amount of practical knowledge about how lives go. They maintain the discipline of naturalistic observation, now largely disowned elsewhere in medicine, experiencing patterns which reveal that not only the biological but also unconscious and interpersonal worlds have their own empirically describable laws—and of course, their ineffable mysteries.

Perhaps most important is the analysts' example of self-development through a required personal psychotherapy, which has ceased to be the norm in psychiatry generally.

I could easily fashion further such statements about any of our knowledge bases: psychiatric wisdom is not family systems theory; it is not neuroscience, and so on. True, the experience of practicing from each of these points of view makes a unique contribution to the whole. But to find our wisdom we need to go beyond these bodies of knowledge, into our interactions with our patients.

To illustrate, I will describe two patients I might see in any given week whose situations superficially appear to be opposites, but for whom the *psychiatric* intervention required of me is essentially the same.

The first is a middle-aged man seen at a rural public clinic. His complaint is "bad nerves," and endless trials of psychotropic medications by family doctors and psychiatrists have failed to quell the patient's anxiety and headaches. Increasingly desperate, he still has high hopes for the next pill.

Twenty minutes of inquiry into the patient's family situation reveals that his elderly father, who had abused him in childhood, is now unable to care for himself and making ever more demands on his son. The patient's rage and guilt, when verbalized, not only make his symptoms comprehensible to me but also introduce to this intelligent but psychologically naive man the novel idea that "bad nerves" can be an expression of conflict and that talking about these connections can be helpful to him. He accepts a referral for therapy.

The second case involves a younger woman seen in my urban private practice, for whom an endless round of psychotherapies, alternative treatments of various sorts, self-help books, and weekend spiritual retreats have only added another layer to her chronic depression: the shame of failure, of flunking out of the joyous New Age.

A straightforward biologically oriented interview reveals the well-known "hysteroid dysphoria" pattern of hypersomnia, rejection sensitivity and craving for sweets—a pattern which classically responds to a particular class of medications, the MAO inhibitors. [These older drugs are now rarely used because of potentially hazardous side effects but remain of theoretical interest.]

So strong is her shame that I will not risk broaching the subject of any kind of antidepressant with her until we have a stronger alliance. For now at least I am able to make sense of some of her behavior patterns as responses to her own depression rather than moral flaws, and she finds this helpful.

What was the *psychiatric* intervention in these two cases? Not the specific technical inquiries, which were different in each case. Not these, but the freeing of each patient from the particular myth of transformation within which he or she was locked—imprisoned by someone's theory and isolated from real help.

The tiresome fact that psychiatrists are therapists of last resort holds one unique advantage: We see everyone else's treatment failures. In general, these other practitioners from whom we tend to inherit our patients are identified with one theory or worldview. The internist represents high-tech Western biomedicine; the psychologist (usually), some particular school of psychotherapy; the holistic practitioner, one or several "alternative" cosmologies; the co-dependency therapist, the Recovery Movement; etc.

In psychiatry we have access to many theories, including all of the above, but what truly drives us is an awareness of our patients' desperation. The wisdom of our greatest teachers has been practical—the wisdom of what works, and even more importantly of: What if nothing works? The wise psychiatrists I have known use their knowledge bases well but lead with their own selves which are both cultivated and spontaneous. They achieve a certain exhilarating freedom from theories, technologies, prescriptions, and "answers" because they are grounded in a tradition of therapeutic intimacy, a collaborative human process based not just on seeing or hearing but most fundamentally on touching (even if there is no physical touching) in a way that only medical work can be.

In other words, psychiatric wisdom is the wisdom of good primary-care medicine. In asserting this medical identity we do not need to apologize for ourselves or ape the other medical specialties with their emphasis on technology and control. We need instead to exemplify, alongside the family practitioners, the fact that good medicine is based as much on relationship as on biology; to help actively define just what medical wisdom is.

A psychiatric Ecclesiastes might say that to every therapy there is a season and a time to every purpose under heaven: a time to listen and a time to talk; a time to interpret and a time to act; a time for unconscious and a time for ego; a time to trust the healing power in a patient's intrinsic process, and let it develop; and a time to waken to its destructive potential and try to abort it.

Through all these seasons, by way of compass, he would remind us of our central task as physicians. That task is *not* the resolution of conflicts, the airing of "issues," the righting of chemical imbalances, the forging of a higher consciousness, the revision of immature defenses, or the articulation of a concept of health—though at times any and all of the above may be involved. Whether cure is possible or not, the doctor's primary aim is ultimately the *relief of symptoms*, which grounds our work in compassion from the beginning. We are always brought home to symptoms, whether hearing them or suppressing them, bargaining with them, or routed by them. We return with our patients to the symptom, that representative of a radically separate, ultimately unknowable Nature (albeit human nature). In the encounter with the Otherness of the symptom we find our truth.

G E T T I N G   M A C I E
O F F   T H E   M O U N T A I N

People don't always want you to do what they ask you to do. I conclude this section and this book with a cautionary tale from my days in the hills of East Kentucky. It portrays in a dramatic way a situation which occurs in more subtle fashion in therapists' offices when we wander naievely in to pre-existing, powerful "family systems." For this reason, though it is a medical doctor's misadventure, I include it in my collection of essays on psychotherapy.

"Macie" was my first published psychiatric piece. Written in 1985, it appeared in the 1988 anthology *Psychiatric House Calls*, edited by John Talbott (American Psychiatric Press).

In the late summer of 1980 I was not yet a psychiatrist but a fledgling general practitioner just out of internship with a penchant for doing the "right thing." My Public Health Service commitment had led me to the south-central Appalachian coalfield, a land as rich in moral ambiguity as it once was in minerals. Lessons awaited me there.

My wife first heard of Macie Slone. The older Slone boy, Jack, came to her clinic with his Californian wife, Lisa. My wife, a physician's assistant with some time to listen, saw Lisa for a sore throat. Soon Jack was invited in, and the sore throat was forgotten while the whole Slone situation poured forth. Jack was a nationally known painter. Despite his mountaineer's appearance and speech, he had made his home in San Francisco since Lisa had "rescued" (her word) him from his mother, Macie, a few years before.

Lisa had been a footloose young artist at the time, searching, she said, for her romantic image of Appalachia. She found it personified in Jack—handsome, talented, and of few but significant words—at a regional craft show. She fell in love, but there was an unexpected problem: Jack couldn't leave home. He would slip out on some pretext to get to occasional craft

131

shows, but that was as far as he ever went. He and his younger brother, Jeff, were in the thrall of a mother who had "not been right" since their father died years before. She regarded her grown sons alternately as her "possessions" or as helpless infants and did not want them out of her sight. The world was full of enemies who aimed to kill her family and take away her land—a hundred acres of remote mountain country. Lisa remembered that, as Jack told his story, his point of view seemed to waver as if part of him accepted his mother's logic. For two years the brothers had lived in isolation, going off the mountain only to get essential supplies while their mother was sleeping, and otherwise living off the land. Jack found time to paint in the winter. He ventured out to shows to secure the family's only income, while Jeff stayed behind making excuses for his brother's absence.

Perhaps the fairy-tale quality of it all hardened Lisa's resolve. After several trips to the shack on the mountain, she managed to induce Jack to run away with her, but she recalled having to lead him by the arm. His talent, her connections, and a current vogue for his particular style led to a measure of success and recognition on the West Coast. Every summer they would return to the shack above Long Creek, but Jeff and Macie had become a self-sustaining system; the new couple found themselves unable to influence it.

Jack had decided that this summer would be different. His brother was nearly thirty, his life in childlike suspension. Attempts to discuss a change with Macie had resulted in her trying to stab Jack with a kitchen knife a couple of times when she thought he was asleep. She was not about to leave the mountain or consider taking medication. If Jeff left, he was afraid she would starve to death or burn herself up fumbling with the rusted-out coal stove. Jack had hidden the guns and large knives but, needless to say, remained uneasy. Macie had to be taken care of.

Local values did not support interference with family situations, whether the problem was violence or some more subtle form of oppression. Gunshot wounds, often resulting from family disputes, were all-too-common emergency room fare. Even when such matters were brought to court they were rarely punished. There were no police outside the larger towns, just a few far-flung sheriff's deputies. No real system for involuntary commitment to a hospital (such as my wife and I had been used to) existed.

On his own, Jack obtained a commitment form, which in Kentucky required two physician signatures. Old Dr. Strout, a local man who had been making house calls for forty years and cared little for public opinion, had been willing to go up to see Macie and sign the papers for twenty dollars. The other doctors around had refused unanimously, either pleading that they were too busy or openly saying that they were wary of repercussions.

The physician's assistant knew someone who might be willing to get involved.

Little shacks punctuated the Long Creek road every so often, and it was by counting them that we found the correct plank bridge across to the

Slone's hollow. Little-used tire ruts beside a smaller creek twisted steeply up to the shack. That morning was clear and fine; the Slones' domain of hillside fields enveloped us. From quite a distance we could see sheets of paper in many of the house's windowpanes. Closer, they appeared to have lines of writing and large, perhaps astrological, symbols on them.

Jack and Lisa rose from the porch to greet us and tell us what to expect. Macie would "see" us as neighborhood children visiting to play and would treat us well if we didn't try to insist we were anything else.

She sat in a rocker facing the coal stove, defying all caricatures: beautiful in her way, beaming, tough as gristle, a seventy-year-old mountain woman in a homespun dress. Jack introduced my wife and me by name. "Come on in, young'uns'," I recall her saying. "I love the young 'uns'." Jeff, a younger, paler shadow of Jack, sat on a couch nearby. We joined him and the others found chairs. Macie rocked, smiled, and chewed her tobacco, speaking to us in half-intelligible phrases with an occasional whistle or snatch of a song. Psychiatric training has since taught me a lot of standard words to impoverish my description of her speech. "Perseveration" comes to mind. But that word, for example, does not convey the quality of calm that Macie projected to the room and beyond, to the land outside the windows. Her perseveration was like that of ocean waves, and like waves her phrases would break with a hiss each time she spat her tobacco juice at the hot stove.

Although we said very little, Macie gradually sensed that this was some sort of inquisition. Sudden angry glances alternated with her former serenity, becoming more frequent until she rose in a huff and stamped out of the room. She returned with a handprinted, badly spelled book, which she gave to me to read. It was far more intelligible than her spoken phrases, purporting to be a "deed" that granted her "sole and rightful possession of my sons, Jack and Jeff, until their deaths," all of the land thereabouts, and all the plants and animals and minerals above, on, or under it. The volume ran to some length because each item was described in detail, right down to parts of plants (e.g. "...and the smooth stem of it is also mine"). Macie then produced a map of the Slone land in her own hand with odd little details about particular trees or bits of landscape. Although geographically accurate, it greatly exaggerated the actual extent of the family's property, according to Jack.

Jack showed us the rest of the little house and the signs in the windows that were "spells" on the land and potential intruders. Macie became thoroughly angry, although she stayed in her chair. Jeff simply looked afraid. I signaled that I had seen enough, and we went outside.

I read the commitment paper and tried to fit all that I'd just seen into a medical judgment. It came down to Macie or Jeff, and Jack assured me that Jeff wanted out. Given that, I read the paper again and it seemed right to sign it. Now Jack could call the sheriff and hope he cooperated. Cash was low, so Jack and Jeff paid me in potatoes. That might have been the end of it.

Several days later I got a call from Jack asking for "advice" on handling the sheriff. His mother was strong and obstinate; handcuffs were a likely eventuality. Jack hated to see this happen to Macie. Did I know any good way to persuade her to go?

In those days, not having had the benefit of a psychiatric education, I didn't tend to worry about legal or ethical ramifications. I just did what seemed right. What seemed right for me, the compassionate young general practitioner, was to offer to go up the hollow with a syringe and get Macie off the mountain in comfort. Jack thought it sounded like a good idea, probably because it had been his idea all along.

It had been raining hard since morning and by the time we got to the Slone's bridge, Long Creek was just a couple of feet below the planks. I hadn't had any success among the local people recruiting help for this expedition; it was the only time they ever disapproved openly of anything I did. Finally Rich, a burly but gentle intensive care nurse from North Carolina, agreed to go with me. We brought two syringes with 100 mg. of thorazine [a powerful old-time antipsychotic] each, a defibrillator, and some emergency medication. An ambulance followed us at a cautious distance, its crew having made it clear that they would not enter the house until Macie was subdued. The twin tire ruts gushed water on our headlights as if the mountain itself were bleeding.

Jack stood with his head down on the porch and said nothing. We all went in and tried to play "young 'uns" again for awhile, but Rich's nursing whites had Macie suspicious from the first. After a few of her searing glances, she retreated to the kitchen. The five of us—Jack, Jeff, Lisa, Rich, and myself—regarded each other as a strange inertia descended on us. I was out of my depth, but Rich had had some state hospital experience and finally went to join Macie in the kitchen. She could tell what he was trying to do and started yelling when she caught sight of the syringe.

I had earlier gotten Jack to promise his and Jeff's active help in this attempt. Now he and his brother stood there, not moving, looking at Rich and me with a sudden fierceness. We began to fear for ourselves. Lisa took them each by the arm, imploring, "You've got to help them!"

"Ambivalence" is another nice psychiatric word. I remember thinking at the time, in a detached way, that only the human being could be in such conflict as to be frozen in the middle of a situation. Then I recalled the gray squirrel in front of an oncoming car, two-thirds of the way across the road, unable to decide whether to get across or go back the way he came. He knows where he *was*, and often as not he'll try to go back there, getting himself killed in the process.

We were two-thirds of the way into this now. Lisa distracted the two brothers while I sat frozen on the couch. Only Rich had the strength to continue. He somehow got behind Macie, emptied one of the syringes, then wrapped his legs around her and fell back on a chair. Macie fumed and thrashed while he spoke to her in soothing North Carolina tones. They remained locked in this fool's embrace while the ambulance idled outside in the rain, until Macie fell asleep.

Rich and I followed the ambulance back down to the Long Creek road, listening to the beat of the wipers and feeling like assassins. There must have been a better way; the sheriff would have done at least as well as we had. Jeff stayed in the shack with Lisa, quietly sobbing, while Jack rode in the ambulance with his mother. We later heard that Macie was awake and out of her restraints by the time they reached the creek mouth. Jack sat across her legs for the remainder of the twisty four-hour trip out to the state hospital.

Jack and Lisa stopped by a few months later. Jeff had joined them in San Francisco and was doing well. They were down to arrange Macie's transfer to a local boarding home and all seemed pleased with the situation. Macie had responded nicely to medication and also to treatment for her previously undiscovered diabetes. They described taking her out to lunch at McDonald's: her fascination, her bold investigation of a world outside herself she had never seen. Their account likened her reactions to a young child's, for whom the mundane fast-food restaurant might as well be Oz.

In 1982 I entered psychiatric residency and have since been involved with perhaps a hundred cases of involuntary hospitalization. None affected me so deeply as Macie's, which I experienced without the insulation of theories, techniques, and diagnostic labels. To have experienced getting Macie off her mountain *naively*, before my psychiatric education, paradoxically exposed me more deeply to the emotional dilemma that psychiatrists face.

As agents of change we must first appreciate the patient's world. Once this work of appreciation has begun, we recall that we are asked to alter, sometimes even destroy, that which we have just begun to understand. We cannot even rely on the patient or family who asked us there to be our steadfast allies; they battle with themselves in asking. We may find ourselves alone with a decision to make, like the squirrel in the middle of the road.

The end of a world causes great pain, however painful that world may have been. I've never been so sure about the "right" thing to do since we got Macie off the mountain.

PART IV:
STILL CARVING, NIGHT AND DAY

INTRODUCTION TO PART IV

If our work isn't about listening to and taking care of people, then it is nothing at all.

A depressed ex-convict tells of the 23 days he spent in solitary confinement after leading a prison riot. Lying on a bare concrete floor in a narrow shaft of light, he is visited by an ant in search of bread crumbs. He amuses himself by making the ant walk back and forth between two hands that dam its progress, and rewards it with the crusts he has not eaten himself. The ant (or one like it) visits the shaft of light daily. It keeps the prisoner alive.

A demented elderly woman on a hospital ward has been ravished by an hallucinatory stallion. She expresses guilt and violation, but there is excitement as well: she is pregnant with a centaur.

The psychiatrists who heard these two recent stories could have done many things to care for these patients, but had they not first listened, their interventions would have been less likely to heal. The human psyche demands to be met on its own terms, seen first in all its irrepressible creativity, before it even temporarily yields to our will. It resembles bamboo, which can be cut back but always finds a way to spring up again.

Our surest source of contact with this psyche is an ever-renewing one: clinical material like that above, if not always so dramatic—images, dreams, feelings, urgent declarations, painful admissions—that is gifted to those of us who work directly with ill, suffering, and conflicted individuals. And as the work of digesting this magma from the inside proceeds, patients and doctors alike must negotiate unprecedented and continually changing social contexts on the outside. Together we witness powerful cultural forces that impinge on the therapeutic relationship, and the very nature of the self. At times, we do their bidding; at others we try to resist them.

Meanwhile the intellectual disciplines entrusted with psyche have proceeded on separate paths that lead away from the perilous richness of the everyday clinical encounter.

Mainstream academic psychiatry and its allied fields are busy vanquishing target symptoms without regard to whether or not any personal meanings may be hidden therein. Protocols for correct (meaning: socially adaptive) thinking have taken over psychiatry's psychotherapeutic arm. And medication, of course, otherwise rules the roost; the sometimes inconvenient psychological questions its use raises going largely ignored.

Psychoanalysis, on the other hand, is fast becoming a branch of literary academe: witness the well-established Freud and Jung industries, the up-and-coming Lacan industry, and so on. In England, I am told, one can even get a diploma in "Psychoanalytic Studies" with the caveat that it does not entitle the diplomate to see patients. What, I wonder, does such training prepare one for? More scintillating cafe conversation? As a clinical treatment in this country, analysis "proper" has long been the intersubjective domain of a privileged few. It has given us an interesting set of heuristics, perspectives from which to listen to our patients, but no usable, provisional consensus about what to do with them in the more typical, attenuated context of contemporary mental health treatment.

I have been arguing for the last decade for the legitimacy of analysis improper: psychodynamic clinical psychiatry, a flexible and pragmatic discipline that need not accept an intellectual status subordinate to that of psychoanalysis. If concepts like the Unconscious, transference, defense mechanism, archetype, holding environment and so on are to survive, if any consensus about their application in mental health treatment is to emerge, psychodynamic psychiatry, not psychoanalysis, will be the reason why. Ideas that emerge directly from the everyday caregiving encounters we have with psyche embedded in culture are as valid as those that come by way of the couch, and, at this point in history, of more pressing social relevance.

The goose is still frozen in the lake, and we are still trying to thaw it out.

• • • • •

On reflection, I realize that my choice to begin the introduction to this final section of my book with the story of my patient, the ex-convict, and his ant visitor came out of a distant but perceptible identification with him. Of course, I have not been living on dried-out bread in an isolated cell, but at times my professional work and particularly my writing has felt like a kind of solitary confinement, with only the restless vitality of my daily visitors, my patients, to sustain me. I know from the correspondence I have had with many other clinicians who have kept faith with the psychiatry they were taught that this feeling has been pervasive among us.

After I published the first edition of this book in 2000, I assumed that I would soon give up writing about my work. Instead (as often happens when a preconceived goal is abandoned) I found that I had a lot more I wanted to say. Much of that subsequent spurt of writing is collected here in Part IV. By the end of it, having despaired again of having any meaningful impact on the contemporary behavioral health care juggernaut, I really did quit. Then, to my surprise, a pro forma inquiry to The Analytic Press yielded an invitation to reissue *The Thaw* with the following, additional material. I was glad that my recent writing would have a wider audience, but even happier to have been encouraged, by this fine publisher's recognition, to keep on writing more.

Lewiston, Maine
3/22/02

141

Is American Psychiatry
Terminally Ill?

Paul Stepansky of The Analytic Press invited me to open this section of more recent essays with an older one, my very first published in *Psychiatric Times* (June 1993). He recognized it as the testament of a psychiatrist whose professional identity had "hit bottom." It was only the large response from similarly despairing practitioners around the country that encouraged me to continue making what had seemed at the time like a lone cry in the wilderness (and that emboldened *Psychiatric Times* to offer me a spot as a regular columnist). I still keep a folder full of letters from psychiatrists responding to this piece.

Rereading it from this distance, I am struck by the fact that most of the themes I have written about since are sounded here and that American psychiatry today is much the same, only more so. The sexual boundary-violation scandals have died down, but hardly disappeared. There is even more emphasis on medicalization and standardized, purportedly "evidence-based," psychotherapies. While the Decade of the Brain did give research neuroscientists a much fuller appreciation of the complexity of the mind-body connection, much clinical practice remains back at the "chemical imbalance" level of understanding.

On the other hand, an alternative consensus still survives among therapeutically oriented psychiatrists like my readership—more than I might have guessed. Squabbles among the "schools" of therapy have very much lessened as it becomes clear that flexible pragmatism is the only viable option for us.

Of all the young psychiatric residents-in-training I have supervised, Dave has a special raw talent. Though he can be vague and tentative, he has two attributes that set him apart. He has a gift for helping patients express the truth about themselves, and he has the ability to offer everything he can to them without promising to offer more.

Dave recently returned from a rotation in England, and has six months left before he graduates and moves away. He has resumed working with the woman patient to whom we now listen on audiotape. During the past year and a half, they have forged a relationship that has benefited them both and helped her begin to emerge from a personal history of tragedy and abuse. With her permission I have been privileged to listen in on the mysterious alchemy that psychotherapy, even in today's hostile climate, still can be.

Dave's instinct has led him to offer his patient a more intensive course of therapy—at the nowadays unheard-of rate of two sessions per week—despite the risk both acknowledge of greater pain after his imminent departure. She has accepted, and now he brings "a sense of urgency" to our supervision session. The best "treatment plan" he has been able to develop consists simply of "saying good-bye"; should he be trying to do something more?

Beneath the surface question of whether he should be throwing more technique, more procedures or interpretations her way, he is feeling me out on an opposite concern. Is he already too involved? As he readily recognizes, his responses on today's tape belie the loss he is feeling, in advance, of this important learning relationship, this tangible human contact which he is likely to remember and draw upon for the remainder of his professional life. Is it ethical of him to consider these feelings of his own in deciding to offer her more?

As he describes his quandary and I try to respond, an invisible audience of experts and interested parties enters the room: malpractice lawyers, training directors, managed-care insurance coordinators, peer reviewers, psychotherapy researchers, ethics committee members, muckraking journalists. They whisper of clinical imprecision, low cost-effectiveness and boundary violations. Yet, I find myself defending his instincts and "treatment plan" regardless of their disapproval. As I do so, I am led again to contemplate the sorry state of my profession.

In 1993, American psychiatry as I have known it is moribund. Despite the continuing clinical skill, compassion and courage of many individual practitioners, and despite impressive scientific advances, the profession as a whole seems to have lost its integrity; it is a rotting ship. When I entered the field 10 years ago from general practice, it was still possible to imagine a career in the independent practice of psychotherapy-oriented psychiatry. Today's new residency graduates have no such illusions. Dave knows he will be hard put to find a setting where he can do the kind of open-ended, individualized work I am teaching him to do. That being the case, our supervision often seems a sentimental anachronism, like the training of modern merchant marine cadets on square-rigged sailing ships because someone thinks it will be good experience, even though they'll be steering oil tankers for a living.

My own trade paper, the American Psychiatric Association's *Psychiatric News*, makes regular pronouncements that private practitioners like myself are, like the spotted owl, headed for extinction along with our old-growth habitat, the office-based, therapy-centered practice where it is still possible to innovate collaboratively with the patient and to ensure his or her complete privacy. An ever-shrinking minority is in full-time private practice, as demand flags and resident recruitment plummets. Many colleagues are looking at alternative careers.

The most important reasons for psychiatry's demise, I believe, are internal to the profession. My view contrasts with the statements of official spokespersons, who tend to focus on external pressures affecting the profession.

There are, indeed, plenty of external pressures: shrinking insurance reimbursements; "managed care" and its intrusions into patient's privacy; and competition with legions of non-medical and nontraditional psychotherapists. Even the prescribing of psychotropics is no longer secure as the sole prerogative of psychiatrists. Family doctors write most antidepressant prescriptions today, and the Ph.D. psychologists with whom they often collaborate are pushing hard for their own prescribing privileges. Our APA's attempts to lobby against the psychologists' drive, often blatantly obvious in their defense of psychiatrists' professional and financial turf, have backfired, serving to highlight our confused identity. The average American still does not know the difference between a psychiatrist and a psychologist. Ironically, we have reinforced the idea that the only difference is that psychiatrists can prescribe. The value of our medical training not only as an education in clinical sciences, but also as an intimate initiation into the human mysteries of birth, healing, illness and death—something no graduate-school seminar can provide— is thereby trivialized.

Among well-educated individuals (such as our fellow physicians), we have become therapists of last resort. The feeling of failure at "having to see a psychiatrist" is often palpable at a first-time visit while positive potentials for growth and healing are nowhere to be found.

One reason for the new patients' dismay is our profession's public image. There has always been a mixture of idealization and mistrust attached to "doctors of the mind" who are privy to people's most secret needs and madnesses. But today the balance has swung so far to the negative side—the cannibal-psychiatrist Hannibal Lecter in *Silence of the Lambs* being the foremost example—that APA has actually hired publicists and mounted a campaign to try to dig us out of the hole.

It would be one thing for a healthy profession to fend off these external threats. But psychiatry's current difficulty in credibly advocating for itself and in attracting vocal allies reveals an organism whose immune system is compromised by a more fundamental and widespread illness. In fact, fiction in its portrayal of loose ethics and irresponsibility is sometimes hard put to improve upon real events within the psychiatric community.

Most visible, for obvious reasons, have been the nationally reported scandals involving psychiatrists and their patients, such as that of former APA president Jules H. Masserman and that of Margaret Bean-Bayog.

Taken as an aggregate, these episodes have stuck to our profession like a collective disgrace, and a *Time* cover story. They are plausible when compared to the evidence one gives most credence to, the statistics closer to home. At any given time, I have one, and sometimes two, patients in my practice who have had some sort of sexual contact with a previous therapist, often a psychiatrist. And over the past few years, I can think of three psychiatrists who have had their licenses suspended for this reason. In a national survey in 1987, 6.4 percent of more than 1,300 psychiatrists surveyed anonymously admitted to having had sexual contact with one or more patients.

Nor is the feeling of betrayal limited to sexual matters. In 1991, for example, Martin Orne, psychiatrist for several years in the 1960s to the poet Anne Sexton, who suicided in 1974, released transcripts of their therapy sessions to the poet's biographer, Diane Wood Middlebrook. While his motives may have been defensible, the effect on the popular perception of psychiatry is an impression that the privacy of the therapy hour is not inviolable, but subject to the needs and wishes of the psychiatrist.

To a public watching with varying amounts of interest, the specifics of events like these are less important than the blurred image of a profession which cannot be trusted. To those of us who daily put our sincere best efforts into this work, each new revelation comes as one more demoralizing kick in the stomach, one more obstacle to building or maintaining trust with our patients.

A second reason for the popular suspicion of psychiatry seems far removed from these intimate betrayals and has instead to do with our increasing and much-vaunted identification with biomedical science. Public mistrust of the "medical model" approach persists despite the amazing, almost science-fiction-like advances made in recent years by the neurobiological wing of psychiatric research. Sophisticated imaging techniques, rapid progress in neurotransmitter biochemistry and such highly effective new drugs as fluoxetine (Prozac) and clozapine (Clozaril) have gained much publicity and attention. But with them, reinforcing the public's wariness, have come controversial reports of "Prozac suicides" and "Halcion murder."

Part of the problem here is endemic in all of medicine: the fact that academic scientist/researchers are operating at a remove from the realities of clinical practice. Their well-designed studies with carefully selected patients have limited relevance to the complex and refractory cases with whom most of the subsequent disasters occur. These occur when some unfortunate clinician has heard genuine claims made for the latest drug and then prescribed it for someone who has not responded well to *any* previous drug, will not respond to this one, and will likely go on defeating such simplistic attempts at cure.

There are conditions and patients that respond to straight-forward pharmacologic intervention, for which the "chemical imbalance" model provides a good approximate understanding. But most psychiatric problems result from complex interactions of inherited biological vulnerability, life history and recent circumstance and cannot be reduced to this simple model which too many self-described "biological psychiatrists" offer their patients instead of taking time to explain more fully (or perhaps to think it through for themselves). This pattern is, in part, understandable in that much of the literature they read elevates the chemical correlates of psychiatric illness to causes.

But the deeper problem is that many psychiatrists, especially newly trained ones, have had little exposure to other ways of looking at their patients' situations. This state of affairs is not likely to improve, as training in psychotherapy—wherein generations of psychiatrists have learned that symptoms sometimes mean something, and that relationships have the power to affect the human psyche for good or ill—is on the wane in residency training. And the most concrete experiential lesson of all, personal therapy for the trainee, "can no longer be considered a requirement for all residents" according to a recent official pronouncement.

I do not mean to suggest that all psychiatrists should be psychotherapists, or that all patients need therapy. Rather, I am saying that a psychiatrist who has never been exposed to the disciplined exploration of another person's subjective experience is doomed to practice in a two-dimensional way regardless of the context. (I shudder to think of the effect this policy will have on the future frequency of exploitative psychiatrist–patient relationships.)

The only kind of psychotherapy that still thrives within the psychiatric fold, aside from a few urban enclaves of psychoanalysis, is the "scientific" kind: standardized, usually short-term approaches that lend themselves to the sorts of outcome of studies whose methodology has been borrowed from the drug research: active treatment, placebo treatment, control group and so on. And like the new drugs, they seem to be highly effective in the academic setting. However, while these "manual-driven" therapies may provide a useful focus and a safeguard against gross incompetence, they do not begin to be adequate for the sorts of human situations most practicing clinicians routinely face. An entire literature is being bred based on the doomed notion that standardized, rather than individualized, psychotherapy, is the most effective.

The "cookbook" mentality of the *DSM-III-R* is now being extended by APA's publication of a series of "treatment guidelines" for such decontextualized symptomatic syndromes such as "major depressive episode" and "panic disorder." These guidelines threaten to stifle creative and original work by clinicians whose patients fit these descriptions. We may soon have to justify deviations from APA-declared "appropriate" treatment to insurers and case reviewers.

In fact, the remedicalization of psychiatry has been one of APA's public relations strategies for years. In order to overcome the stigma we are heirs to, we have been exhorted to become "more like other doctors," more scientific. Granted, a measure of scientific rigor may have been a necessary antidote to an earlier generation's excesses in fitting reality to the theoretical dogmas of psychoanalysis. But the current push, engineered by academic psychiatrists who have never practiced general medicine, is based on a narrow idea of what science and medicine are.

Any useful medical science has to include the kind of naturalistic observations that come from knowing individual personalities over time. Statistical generalizations can cancel out just those exceptions to the overall pattern which are most important for us to understand. But alas, anything unquantifiable is today consigned to the realm of the "anecdotal" and "uncontrolled" and disowned as legitimate information. Ironically, psychiatrists often have to look outside their own field—to the writings of the neurologist Oliver Sacks, for example—for role models in achieving this kind of understanding.

In its quest to remedicalize, then, psychiatry has ended up making itself spiritually poorer. It has imitated just those aspects of the dehumanizing pseudo-objectivity that has alienated so much of the public from medicine in general, rather than focusing on our unique and humanizing contributions to medicine: the understanding of individuals over time; the tradition of healing in relationship. This emphasis has sent our patients flocking to other practitioners in search of just these capacities. The tactic has even failed with the "other doctors," who have followed the patients elsewhere. They no longer refer patients, as a rule, unless they anticipate some psychopharmacologic treatment beyond their own capabilities; the well-motivated patients in search of psychotherapy are generally sent to non-medical therapists.

Most telling of all, it is the Ph.D. psychologists who are usually hired to teach the "behavioral medicine" curricula (even the word "psychiatry" is unwelcome) in family practice and primary-care internal medicine residencies. Primary care physicians seek ways to understand their patients, not just classify and medicate them.

The polarity upon which American psychiatry has foundered can be expressed with one overused word: "boundaries." On the one hand there are the problems of unclear boundaries between psychiatrist and patient, typified in the extreme by sexual liaisons. On the other we have nothing *but* boundaries, walls built of medical tests, scans, diagnostic labeling and cookbook treatment that all but preclude contact. What these seeming opposites have in common is an unconscious attachment to power and control.

Psychiatrists are confronted daily with the human condition of solitary helplessness, pain and loss—a condition which in other times and places has been the province of trusted elders or religious leaders. The great psychiatric educator Elvin Semrad recognized this when he once observed that "psychiatry is the only branch of medicine which asks patients to bear their pain." Teachers like him have gotten harder to find in the course of a contemporary psychiatric education. His was the traditional wisdom born of experience with not knowing and not being able to control, and he sought to help above all by sharing honestly in the existential conditions of his patients' lives. Whatever (necessarily imperfect) technical assistance could be provided would have that sharing at its base.

Today's psychiatrists are schooled not in wisdom but only in knowledge and control. We must discover our helplessness for ourselves, or remain unconsciously "above it," with no basis for meeting the helplessness our patients experience. Our training has taught us to build conceptual castles in the air to defend ourselves from our patients' pain, and our own. In like manner, the two poles above follow this pattern. The diagnostic expert with categories, tests and pills seeks to "master" the pain with science; the therapist seeks to become a perfect nurturer, able to "reparent" the regressed patient and grandiosely to know what he or she needs to internalize ("I'm your mommy and I love you very much" said one of Margaret Bean-Bayog's flash cards for Paul Lozano).

Either case taken to its logical extreme finds only one person in the room: the psychiatrist, pursuing his or her own agenda at the expense of an objectified patient. The possibility of real human contact is lost, even if the pair becomes "intimate." Seen in this light, the movie image of Dr. Hannibal Lecter preying upon his patients ceases to be mere specious slander, best ignored, and becomes instead a meaningful nightmare with a diagnostic message for us.

I told Dave that his treatment plan, far from providing an inadequate goal, seemed to me to contain an admirable overarching purpose: A good-bye that we are powerless to avert is written into all real relationships. If Dave steers a middle course wherein human contact remains possible, keeping his own emotional stake clearly in view, he is likely to avoid the positions of "scientist" or "lover," which are both misnomers. He and his patient will make a good good-bye: to each other and to childhood; to forever; to the dream of a life without pain and death; to the idea of complete fulfillment in a dependent relationship. They will have experienced together the real conditions of life on this killing floor, and both of their own lives will be enriched thereby.

Dave's sense of urgency, I feel, is not just about his patient's therapy, but about the fate of the profession he has entered. My rhetorical title notwithstanding, psychiatry will, of course, survive in some form. Hospital-based clinicians may ultimately become the "sub-specialty of internal medicine" that one of my own teachers envisioned. And someone will need to care for the chronic mentally ill, whose plight society as a whole refuses to acknowledge. (If resident recruitment drops much lower, psychologists wielding prescription pads may need to be called in for this role.) But the collaborative form of experiencing at the heart of psychiatry may soon be gone, and Dave and I may both be making our good-byes to the most rewarding part of our professional lives.

BOUNDARY VIOLATIONS AND
THE FALL FROM EDEN

In this piece I returned to some of the evolutionary issues treated less theoretically in "Raffaela's Hug" (Part II): the notion that therapist burnout (or, as it is now fashionably called, "compassion fatigue") and boundary violations may be evidence not just of individual psychopathology but of a mismatch between our behavioral-genetic inheritance and the world we must inhabit. "Eden" appeared in *Psychiatric Times,* June 2001.

There has been a lot of water over the dam in the past 10,000 years since the beginnings of agriculture and complex urban societies. For the preceding million and a half years, human social organization had been more or less the same. Even while developing upright posture, tools, and language, those species which carried the DNA sequence that defines the hominid line—Australopithecus afarensis, Homo erectus, and finally Homo sapiens—roamed their mostly African ranges in small hunter-gatherer bands thought typically to consist of 20–30 closely related individuals. In this evolutionary context, if you helped someone survive (e.g., shared your food, nursed the injured), you could reasonably expect to get the help back when you needed it. You and your comrade had a history together, and such mutual helping benefited you both, bettering the odds that your own DNA sequence and your friend's (likely very similar) would propagate through time.

Such is the story evolutionary theorists have been telling us for the last 30 years about the origin of mutual helping behavior, or, in their language, "reciprocal altruism," in humans and many other social species. The fulfilling inner experience we helpers have, say these theorists, is epiphenomenal to the calculus of gene propagation; it is a good feeling that simply reinforces the most adaptive behavior just as surely

150

as the "cute response" moves mothers to nurture and protect their off-spring. (The analogous response in mice can be removed by knocking out a gene called fos-B; indifferent mother mice lacking it let their children starve.)

It is no wonder that this story has fallen mostly on deaf ears in the mental health community. Most of us resent having our cherished ideals reduced to organic chemistry, even if we are comfortable wielding chemotherapeutic treatments. And yet, incomplete as it is (and often half-baked, as presented in many popular books), the evolutionary argument, in my experience, casts a revealing light on the personal evolution of many a psychiatrist.

Many of us begin as idealists eager to care for people, but few remain deeply engaged with large numbers of very needy patients after a decade or so. Aside from leaving the profession, there are two adaptive escape routes. (This was equally true before managed care, although the proportion of psychiatrists choosing each has been altered by it.) Both are attempts to survive the overwhelming emotional pain and need in whose path modern society places psychiatrists as specialized professionals expected to deal with it—in exchange for pay and under circumstances wholly unlike those in which our capacity to meet needs and to solace pain developed.

In one typical escape from this overwhelming situation, the established psychiatrist in private practice progressively sets limits on the number and severity of cases he sees. The chaotic borderlines or those with refractory Axis I syndromes are left to the big systems or to the newer private practitioners.

A second escape route, open to academic and institutional psychiatrists, is the retreat into some form of professional detachment. This path appears variously as a theoretical or research orientation, or focus on therapeutic technique, on administrative procedure and systems management, or, more simply, the superficial "med-check" routine.

A third, nonsanctioned escape leads psychiatrists to impairment, addiction, and boundary violations with patients. The last is our main concern here. I argue that it can be seen as a perverse attempt to get reciprocal altruism to really work; to get something tangible back from patients by way of meeting personal needs inappropriately.

At best, experienced psychiatrists, consciously aware of the need to conserve themselves for the long haul, pick and choose where they get deeply involved. Whatever their chosen escape from the undiluted, overwhelming needs of limitless members of patients, they do not turn up their noses at colleagues who have responsibly chosen another. At worst, the private-practice therapists sneer at their institution-based colleagues for overmedicating patients and not listening to them, while the institutional psychiatrists sneer back at the psychotherapists for avoiding the heavy work: large numbers of very difficult patients.

Rarely does either group see a connection between its own choice and that of the third, impaired or boundary-violating group. We quickly distance ourselves from them without so much as a "There but for the grace of God go I." If with unalloyed moralistic denial we deal with our unconscious fear of falling into this quicksand, we label those "fallen" psychiatrists as sociopathic predators. (Of course, a small minority of them are.) Or, if our intellectual defenses have a more sophisticated polish, we may come up with some Kohutian verbiage about grandiose mirror transferences and narcissistic merger. Whatever our preferred explanation, we are steadfastly talking about something that happens to *other* people.

These explanations (particularly the Kohutian verbiage) are not without merit, as far as an understanding of individual psychology is concerned. But they distract us from an incontrovertible fact that both Darwin and Freud, in their different ways, brought to our attention some while back. That is, human beings were not genetically designed to live in the social world in which they now find themselves. Psychotherapy and medicine are among the "helping professions" unknowingly assigned to deal with the personal consequences of this simple fact. By focusing on the *individual* psychopathology of each "fallen" psychiatrist (I use the language of the biblical Eden purposefully here), we neglect the *collective* significance of the phenomena of boundary violation and impairment.

In the modern professionalized situation, the bottom drops out of small-group reciprocal altruism. As isolated and anonymous individuals encounter each other, having little past or future together, two things happen. The first is that, without the support of a true community, the limits of an individual helper's resources are reached sooner and more often. There are not enough helpers to go around. The second is that the help-seeker often brings to each encounter a greater backlog or depth of unmet needs (and depth of frustration if current needs are not met). In this context—on purely Darwinian grounds—"selfless" altruism ceases to be so attractive. Competing and more immediate self-preservation instincts gain a stronger position. The helper often shifts, under their influence, to strategies that are sure, in the near term, to conserve resources: ways of obtaining immediate gratification or discharging uncomfortable affect at the help-seeker's expense. It is in this perverse sense that the helper is trying to make his originally altruistic involvement "deliver" some reciprocal benefit, or at least stop being a drain.

We have become quite skilled at constructing high-minded theoretical rationales for rejecting needy, messy patients. They need to "experience limit-setting," to "develop internal motivation," and so on. It is

for their own good. (Interestingly, some of the more successful innovative treatments for difficult patients, like ACT teams and a more
relapse-forgiving substance-abuse treatment, throw these "compliance"
rationales out the window. They dilute the patients' need through team
approaches and group modalities that recall the hunter-gatherer bands
of yore.) The sense of emotional relief that occurs after "limiting"
patients out of our lives should tip us off that something instinctual,
not just theoretical, is going on.

There is another form of objectification aside from the purportedly
theoretical one of limiting patients out. It leads to exploitation of the help-
seeker for the helper's own gratification. Here, too, boundary-violating
therapists are sometimes found to have constructed quite a coherent
theory about what their patients needed to experience. Most overt
therapist–patient sexual boundary violations occur in this context, but
there are more subtle possibilities as well.

I recall a photograph of a female therapist taken by her male patient
in a playful moment, which was later used in a chronicle of the even-
tual therapeutic disaster. I imagine this therapist luring the damaged
child she saw in her patient and bringing his (and thus her own) playfulness back to life in her misguided efforts to heal him (herself). Again,
this was not true altruism, though it may have seemed like a quintes-
sentially "intimate" experience. The therapist could not follow through,
in real life, on the intimacy that her behavior seemed to promise and
that the unfortunate patient took literally. The devastated patient later
suicided. That each member of this therapeutic dyad may, at the moment
captured by the photograph, have felt wonderfully "close" to the other
obscures the deeper reality that the therapist's behavior was selfishly,
not altruistically, motivated on the level we are describing.

To summarize, there are two opposite modes of objectifying patients
and their needs: "technical" limit-setting (to which, granted, there sometimes is no viable alternative) and boundary-losing "symbiosis." Between
these there is a needle to thread: the hard work of remaining engaged
and distinct. One tries to keep one's boundary, containing and processing one's own evoked affects while maintaining contact with the
patient in order to help him in a parallel process. This very tall order is
the concern of much of the modern psychoanalytic literature.
Successfully done, it *is* altruistic, but the long-term payoffs—money, status, gratitude (these first three are iffy), the exhilaration of mastery—are
far more abstract than the exemplary "hunk of meat" that rewarded our
altruistic forebears for their efforts and presumably helped select their genes
for dissemination.

It is no wonder that we so regularly fall short of this therapeutic
ideal of engaged distinctness. Our behavioral genetics were designed for
the earlier situation and are inadequate for the present one. We are try-

ing to cross the ocean in a cardboard canoe. When we see that it is leaking, there is a strong motivation to jump overboard and swim for shore.

Thus, viewed in the cold light of evolutionary theory, modern psychiatry in both its psychopharmacological and psychotherapeutic aspects is often in the business of making new and better defense mechanisms to help us bearers of the human hunter-gatherer genome to cope with our unprecedented social situation. We psychotherapists, from whose ranks the boundary violators usually come, try to reconstruct an Eden that never was, in which altruism and its accompanying warm feelings can operate unfettered by the context of real community and real participation in one another's lives. There is a regressive longing for the world of the perfectly nurtured child here, which is why speaking of the "fallen" psychotherapist and patient, who act out this longing literally, seems apt. Acted out or not, the psychotherapeutic Eden (as pictured, for example, in the photograph I just recalled) provides a respite from the anonymous, postindustrial culture outside the door, an Eden wherein patient and therapist alike feel heard and seen as persons of individual worth rather than as objects manipulated by market forces.

Meanwhile, psychopharmacology and the more directive sorts of therapy (those which "correct irrational beliefs") are busy building a different kind of Eden in which, if you can't be one of the few at the top of the modern dominance hierarchy, at least you can have (with our assistance) approximately the same balance of neurotransmitters. An SSRI can do this for you directly, or a "corrected" cognitive schema of your place in the world can do it indirectly (but verifiably, according to before-and-after metabolic neuroimaging studies). Or, if society's demands remain beyond reach, perhaps stimulant medication can help you attain a more acceptable level of productivity, with the enhanced security and lifestyle options that accrue to those who can maintain it.

Myths can be life-giving at times, destructive at others. If psychiatry has any remaining potential as a socially progressive force, this Eden is one myth we need to lose. We must awaken from the unconscious thrall it still has over our professional lives in the form of unexamined assumptions and misconceptions about the work we do. In its modern psychiatric and psychotherapeutic versions, the renascent Garden of Eden myth now distracts us from consciously integrating our own discoveries about who we humans really are and how we really got here. It obscures the truths about modern life that impinge equally on those psychiatrists who "succeed" and those whose careers visibly go off course.

As responsible physicians we need, of course, to treat mental disorder, to prescribe medication, to perform psychotherapy. But our interventions are stopgaps, not solutions to the mismatch between our genetics and the culture we live in. Can we practice in such a way as to *enhance* our patients' perceptions about what is really going on in the social world? (Or validate those perceptions? In my experience, many patients see, in their own ways, exactly what is going on.) If not, we will remain in an ironic position: advocates of making the unconscious conscious, even as we unconsciously promise to do the impossible, or worse, act out the Eden myth with our patients.

Only in community does Homo sapiens have any chance of dealing with the evolutionary/cultural mismatch and its ubiquitously unrecognized consequences. We psychiatrists can begin to create community for ourselves as soon as we recognize that we are all fallen psychiatrists in a fallen world.

THERE ARE REALLY ONLY THREE
KINDS OF PSYCHOTHERAPY

In this piece (*Psychiatric Times*, November 2001) I revisited my intermittent hobby of developing a General Theory of Psychotherapy. As I have said, I am always wary of Grand Systems because of the danger that some unsuspecting clinician might mistake them for reality, and so have avoided making a career of spinning such systems. On the other hand, our trainees' ongoing need for some general orientation to a bewildering array of interventions, whose underlying philosophical assumptions are often mutually contradictory, has given me ample excuse to offer occasional overviews like "Getting Two (2.0) People into the Room" in Part II, and like the following.

The mainstream of our profession has ceased paying much formal attention to the help our patients get from the doctor-patient relationship itself. But patients are stubborn. They still expect to have helpful relationships with us! Witness the ill-informed boyfriend of a public-clinic patient who asked me, at the close of a medication visit, "But when is she going to see a *psychiatrist*? She has things to talk about!" Equally disturbing was the well-meaning enthusiasm of a young psychiatrist interviewing for work at the same facility when I told him that I use my psychotherapy training there in many a patient encounter. "Oh, like if there's time you might do a little cognitive therapy on 'em?"

We psychotherapists have ourselves to blame for this state of affairs, having husbanded our subspecialty's development in two narrow directions while psychopharmacology and neuroscience have dramatically broadened their own worldviews. Some of us have manualized and proceduralized psychotherapy (or rather, certain psychotherapies) in imitation of procedural, technology-driven medicine, so as to be good citizens

156

in the world of "indications," "interventions," and "outcomes." Most new psychiatrists have had some exposure to these techniques, but few seem inspired by them.

Another potentially influential group has circled the wagons for psychoanalysis and psychodynamic therapy. The large body of literature this group continues to generate takes many fascinating forms, from the quasi-literary to the quasi-neurological, but few psychiatrists-in-training read it.

Neither of these two currents in psychotherapy convincingly illuminate, or render more effective, our work with the entire spectrum of patients we see in everyday general psychiatric practice.

What sense can we possibly expect our trainees to make of this Tower of Babel? Unless they are unusually persistent they will either stick to the DSM and the meds, or (sometimes *and*) develop their own ways of conceptualizing personality and human nature, often with the help of pop psychology or New Age spirituality. In both cases, this dooms them to repeat sundry mistakes of the past, because an intellectually rigorous psychology of relationship, cognizant of boundaries and power arrangements, is missing. Should those of us who still try to teach psychotherapy in this inhospitable clime simply accept that the next generation will have to reinvent the wheel, or can we do any better for them?

We can, and it isn't all that hard. A global overview of the psychotherapeutic enterprise, based not upon theory but upon what therapists actually do, is easy to provide, and reveals that there are really only three kinds of psychotherapy. I will begin my description with the rather typical odyssey of a real patient at a residency training program.

This patient's prolonged panic attack began when her mother arrived from out-of-state at the local bus terminal in a hospital johnny, seeking her care. Unable to cope, the patient was brought to the ER by her husband. She was so desperately anxious as to admit to suicidal ideation: the "Open sesame!" of our triage culture. At age 31, this secured her first psychiatric hospitalization and evaluation.

The patient settled down quickly with the help of anxiolytics and an alternative placement for her regressed, mentally ill mother. But during her brief stay, an alert inpatient resident noticed that she engaged in several classic compulsive rituals, including much hand-washing and showering. Referral was made for outpatient psychotherapy with another resident, who would obtain supervision in the cognitive-behavioral treatment of obsessive–compulsive disorder in addition to the usual medication trials.

The outpatient resident got more than he'd bargained for. It was difficult for him to concentrate on response-prevention and thought-stopping techniques under the silent, watchful eye of the patient's husband—and she insisted upon his presence "to feel comfortable." The resident kept trying, and one day when the husband had to leave the session early, the patient volunteered that in her own mind, the pervasive sense of "dirtiness" that kept her always washing had something to do with repeated episodes of sexual abuse by her mother in childhood. There was also fear of retribution by mother for "not being a good girl" which transferred in the present to her husband. His idea of good behavior was that she never leave their apartment alone.

It became clear to this intelligent resident that, beyond the illness dimension of Axis I OCD, a relational dimension would have to be entered to treat this patient successfully. A newcomer to the incoherent shipwreck of non-psychopharmacological psychiatry, he understandably groped for some of the remaining scraps of a psychological outlook that are still afloat. Childhood trauma . . . pathological dependence. . . . Axis II borderline personality disorder? Well, close enough to try dialectical behavior therapy (DBT), opined the supervisor.

And so, aided by the husband's periodic departures after check-in, the resident soldiered on with "chain analyses" of anxious thoughts and other such techniques in a DBT-like individual therapy (the skills classes, of course, were unacceptably anxiety-provoking). Eventually the patient stopped coming, and when the resident finally called, she told him that she was afraid she would always be a disappointment to him, and was wasting his valuable time. Could she see the hospital resident who'd originally admitted her "just to talk?"

To the second resident's chagrin, the patient proceeded to settle in comfortably with the original resident, attending regularly although she (the hospital resident) was even more of a therapeutic neophyte and knew no specific techniques. In fact, she said, "I have no idea what I'm doing!" But she is clearly doing something specifically effective for the first goal of any therapy: keeping the patient in the room. The patient is comfortable enough to dispense with the husband's presence. A second "safe place" is emerging which can compete with the safety of the husband's total control, and within which she can begin to take possession of herself.

We can imagine where things might go from here if the utilization reviewers are kept at bay. Perhaps patient and resident (or the resident's successor) will feel ready to retry the response-prevention strategies that failed at first, building on the strength of a working relationship. Or perhaps they will work directly on that relationship itself, when the idealized "safe" therapist inevitably falls from grace and disappoints (or enrages) the patient. Ideally, the patient will eventually work on both behavior and relationship, though not necessarily with the same therapist.

This patient exemplifies the everyday complexity of the real-world population psychiatrists treat. Hers is not a pure form of a DSM-described illness that dutifully improves like the cases in academic studies ("OCD + CBT = OK", "BPD + DBT = OK" etc., as I like to joke).

Table 1: Our Patient's Three-Layer Biopsychosocial cake

Setting	Inpatient unit, ED, CMHC	Outpatient psychotherapy
Bio-	Rapid-cycling bipolar; chronic depression. OCD	Bipolar II; cyclothymia; panic disorder
-Psycho- (personality diagnosis)	Borderline personality disorder	Borderline or narcissistic traits
-Social (historical referent)	PTSD spectrum	"Narcissistic injury"

Source: Genova p (2001)

Instead, she is the usual biopsychosocial layer cake (see Table 1) of Axis I syndrome (bio-), relational disturbance (psycho-), and developmental damage (-social). Because of this, benign power—here, the doctor who tries to do response-prevention—is not a viable reality for her. Before she can get help, she needs help with getting help. And that is what the resident who "doesn't know what she's doing" is giving the patient.

And in the real world of clinical practice, based not on theory but on the unspoken power narrative embedded in therapeutic relationship, there are only three kinds of therapy (see Table 2): supportive, directive, and relational. Our patient began her odyssey in the directive column, where most contemporary psychiatric treatment starts, first with

Table 2: Three Kinds of Psychotherapy

	Supportive	Relational	Directive
Premise	Person centered; technique oriented	Person centered; process oriented	Symptom focused; technique oriented
Power	Expert-object; respite from status quo—"nurturance"	Subject-Subject; subvert status quo—"autonomy"	Expert-object; adapt to status que—"adjustment"
Example	Supportive therapy; self psychology; pharmacotherapy	Psychoanalysis; psychodynamic tx; experiential/Gestalt	CBT, DBT, EMDR; psychoeducation; pharmacotherapy

Source: Genova P (2001)

the CBT, then DBT. When she came back, it was to the supportive column, albeit to a therapist who hadn't yet learned its language. If all goes well, she will finish in the relational column, probably availing herself again of directive techniques along the way.

The underlying premises of each kind of therapy establish a power structure within the doctor–patient relationship; a structure which the doctor may not have thought through in advance, and which he might not endorse if he had. With deliberate exaggeration, therefore, let me explicitly voice the power narrative of each of these three forms of therapy to show the differences between them.

When I speak of power, I refer to the therapist's power to define the nature of reality. Thus, in directive therapies, the unspoken narrative is, "I, the therapist, am powerful and know what is or isn't dangerous [in anxiety disorders], is or isn't negativistic [depression], is or isn't real [psychosis]. I know the diagnosis and causes of your illness and I direct you to change your thoughts/feelings in the following way," etc.

Such a narrative reiterates the existing social status quo and asks the patient to adjust to it. This is often a good and necessary thing, as with a potentially violent paranoid man in the ER, or a widowed woman whose grief has extended into major depression. But because many damaged patients are unable to let themselves be helped by a benign authority —unable, in Winnicott's words, to "use the object"—the directive therapies don't work as often as their academic proponents would like to think.

While the supportive therapies are centered on the person rather than the symptoms, their power narrative has a remarkable underlying similarity to that of their directive cousins. "I, the therapist, am powerful —powerful enough to keep the world at bay. I will create the environment and give you the nurturance that you need. Let yourself unfold under my protection, bask in my empathy," etc.

Instead of actively reinforcing the social status quo, this narrative provides the patient a temporary respite from it. Once again, this is often a good and necessary ("indicated") thing, as in the resident's case presented above. I want to stress, though, that it is a technical approach in that it purports to "know" what is wrong—environmental stresses, developmental deficits from childhood—and to be able to ameliorate or correct it through consciously (even if intuitively) modulated enactments on the part of the therapist. In comparison to directive therapy, the harsh diagnostic language is muffled and there is some implicit faith in an intrinsic healing process which supportive therapy tries, indeed, to support. But the power arrangement in which a knowing therapist administers techniques to a malfunctioning patient remains the same. I maintain that this is even true of Kohutian self psychology, which has developed a rich and beautiful theoretical language to describe its own version of supportive therapy. Such language does not change the fact that the therapist largely defines the nature of reality—an arrangement much more obvious and above-board in the less "humanistically" couched directive therapies. Of course, what experienced practitioners from any well-established "school" of psychotherapy actually do is likely to span all three of the types of therapy in this classification scheme at some time or another; it is only either very new, or very partisan, practitioners who refuse to adapt their behavior to the needs of a reasonable range of patients.

Relational therapy remains to be described, and it is as important not to idealize it as it is not to devalue the other two forms. It does not fit all or even most patients' needs, and its irresponsible application can be not only "contraindicated" but cruel. However, it is the only form of therapy whose power narrative allows both doctor and patient to be subjects engaged in an unpredictable process, rather than an Expert and the object of his technique. "I, the therapist, possess an institutionally sanctioned role as well as education and experience. But my power and knowledge are limited. I offer no more nor less than an honest professional relationship whose primary purpose is to address your problem(s), but through which I fully expect to question myself, learn, and grow as well."

The language of Martin Buber's "I–Thou" dialogue, Jurgen Habermas' "communicative action" and Winnicott's ingenuous term "object use" (which is really about subjects), all aptly describe such a relationship. Therapy takes the form of questions and statements about one's experience of self and other, and its power lies chiefly in the immediate interaction regardless of how much importance the therapist attributes to constructs such as transference, the Unconscious, "developmental issues," the "cycle of experience" (from Gestalt theory), and so on. We all have our favorite constructs, our own ways of skinning a cat.

Because honest reciprocal dialogue fosters autonomy, independent thinking, and acceptance of one's own emotional reality, it is subversive to the social status quo and its usual power arrangement of Expert and object. While patients retain, even improve upon, their ability to get help (including medical care) through relational therapy, its premise encourages them to become the ultimate Experts and Authorities on their own mental and interpersonal lives.

Before I conclude, two important corollaries to this triune scheme deserve mention. First is the place of the powerful modality of group psychotherapy. The various approaches to it fall into the same categories: supportive (peer and professional support groups), relational (process-oriented groups) and directive (psychoeducational and skills groups). As in individual therapy, actual practice favors hybrids rather than pure forms. Family therapies, with which I am less familiar, probably follow analogous patterns.

The other corollary involves the role of medication. It may be directive (as with antipsychotics in acute delusional mania, which aim to change mental content) or supportive (as with temporizing anxiolytics or antidepressants when used to prolong a patient's survival in an intolerable home situation: here the effort is to dull mental content). But medications can never be relational, much as patients sometimes attempt to have relationships with us through them, symbolically mediated by "side effects," paradoxical responses, and refractoriness to treatment. This is one reason why longer visits and individual attention lead to more successful pharmacotherapy.

Giving psychiatric trainees an overview of these three kinds of psychotherapy demystifies the field and helps them to find their place in it. They can then move beyond the procedural "see one, do one, teach one" mentality of medical school. Instead of learning to "do some therapy on 'em" in only standardized ways, trainees will begin to look at their own natural aptitudes, as well as their intrinsic limitations and how possibly to stretch them. Otherwise we consign them to the learning of an ever-narrowing, mechanistic approach to human problems.

RABBI AMONG THE MECHANICS

Having survived the negative publicity generated by the Recovered Memory controversy of the 1980s and early 90s (see "Living with Doubt," Part I), the movement now known as "Trauma-Oriented Psychotherapy" revived itself at the turn of the century, in part with the help of a widely practiced new technique called EMDR (Eye Movement Desensitization and Reprocessing). An encounter with Dr. Paul Ornstein, the distinguished Hungarian-born psychoanalyst and Holocaust survivor, at a training conference provided me the opportunity to reconsider what is most important about recovery from trauma. This article appeared in the May, 2000 *Psychiatric Times*, and Ornstein honored me by writing, "You captured the essence of the day with me beautifully . . . even if I cannot view myself as a Rabbi."

The videotape ends and all the lights go up. About two-thirds of the audience of psychotherapists vigorously applauds the apparently successful conclusion of a taped therapy session, while the rest of us sit in silence. The attractive presenter, an expert in "Eye Movement Desensitization and Reprocessing" (EMDR), has made a few more converts among those enrolled at the trauma conference. Tomorrow her workshop will be full to bursting.

And tomorrow I will sit with a group of eight (two of whom I persuaded to change workshops), listening to an elderly Jewish psychoanalyst with a persistent accent speak and answer questions about his decades of clinical work and how he survived a Nazi slave-labor camp as a young man in World War II Hungary.

After a period of eclipse related to the Recovered Memory/Multiple Personality morass of the late 80s and early 90s, trauma treatment has re-emerged as a hot topic on the mental health scene. Apart from the obvious ubiquity of that which it purports to treat, its popularity within the professional mainstream may be due to the fact that trauma treatment is the last bastion of *story* in contemporary psychiatry. The development of a detailed narrative understanding of the impact of environment and events upon personality has largely been abandoned elsewhere in the field. In trauma treatment, at least clinicians still have a legitimate rationale for listening to stories. Even today, many who choose to enter psychiatry want this experience to be a part of their work.

The problem with early 21st-century trauma treatment is that it too often hears the *same* story.

Let's rewind that EMDR video as an example. The therapist has been working for about a year with a woman, looking to be in her thirties, whose mother tried to choke her as a little girl (among many other things). In this session, the therapist repeatedly brings the patient back to this particular memory. It is a sort of "imaginal exposure" therapy structured by the EMDR procedures (which will not be detailed here), and seems to be a direct descendant of similar techniques whose common features—safe context, sensory focusing, exposure—have long been known to be helpful in treating discrete psychological trauma.

Progressively through the videotaped series of conversations occurring after each "set" of bilateral alternating sensory stimulation, we see undeniable affective change. At first overwhelmed almost beyond words, the patient becomes calmer and more able to reflect verbally on her helpless position. By the end, when she "hears" mother coming up the stairs, she laughs, ridiculing her abuser as if she'd been a cartoon monster: "He-e-ere she comes!"

In a simple polarity reversal, the objectified has become the objectifier. Clearly, the patient feels better, and we learn from the presenter that she conducts herself more effectively with an intimidating co-worker as a result. But there is something missing here. Her own helplessness and her mother's rage are alike recurring experiences attached to the human condition. Simply moving the patient from terror into mockery displaces the dehumanization onto mother. Is not some sort of human understanding (if not necessarily forgiveness) necessary for true healing? Are we doing the patient a favor by leaving her feeling so powerful, or are we fostering denial; depriving her of a unique and useful awareness of human vulnerability that her history might give her?

Whatever particular nuances, even potential sources of strength, that might have existed within this woman's trauma story have been subsumed into the generic Trauma Story, which goes something like this: the old Powerful Other was bad and traumatized you. I am a new, good Powerful Other and I will make *you* powerful (or in EMDR's computerized language, I will "install positive emotional resources").

EMDR is the scientific shamanism of today, as was the Ericksonian hypnosis and "neurolinguistic programming" I eagerly learned in the 1980s, as were Freud and Breuer's abreactive techniques from *Studies in Hysteria* in the 1890s, as were Mesmer's "magnetic passes" in the 1770s. They all worked, some of the time, probably most often with relatively healthy people who had suffered discrete, non-pervasive trauma. The bulk of double-blind studies carefully documented by Eileen Shapiro and her followers involves short-term technical treatment with survivors of catastrophes, natural disasters, rape. By the time our presenter has gotten a year into "EMDR work" with the videotaped patient who suffers from a chronic PTSD syndrome, she is doing relational psychotherapy by another name. I wonder whether her technician's stance will eventually beget a negative transference, and if so whether the cognitive/behavioral/EMDR context will have any room for it, any way to use it well. Or will the patient be "cured" and take what seems to be a stunted, defensive autonomy elsewhere—to another therapist, or to conflictual real-life relationships?

What about the studies? EMDR easily beats "supportive psychotherapy" controls in acute trauma treatment. But does any serious supportive psychotherapy willfully avoid any discussion of traumatic events? And then (hail science!) there are the before and after PET scans, showing increased metabolism in the speech areas after eye movements or alternating sounds have tricked neural activity into crossing the corpus callosum. Would simply engaging the mouth in any well-thought-out way have been equally effective in luring the activity across?

Finally, what about the EMDR partisans' boast that, in short-term treatment comparisons, they shave a session or two off the time other similar methods take to reach the same outcome? Is faster always better? In many conditions, particularly more chronic ones (like obesity), more gradual change holds up better.

Don't get me wrong. When a senior resident, seeking to add to his technical armamentarium, recently asked me whether to learn hypnosis (which I have used) or EMDR, I told him EMDR, precisely because it is more likely to become the technical lingua franca of the day. In the immediate future there will probably be many more people using it with whom he can compare notes than people using hypnosis. And as the latest thing, it will evoke positive expectations from patients. I would be learning it were I at his stage.

But today, as I look back on the successes I had with the Ericksonian techniques I learned, I tend to attribute them to a certain ripeness or readiness on the patients' part more than to my particular method. And with the relationally disturbed patients on the more complex and chronic end of the descriptive category of "PTSD," positive expectations on both sides weren't enough, and any healing achieved was in the context of a painfully negotiated long-term relationship. Techniques sometimes altered the playing field, but never the game. No one says this better than James Gustafson (1995) in *The Dilemmas of Brief Psychotherapy*: "Solution-focused mechanics are only half right. . . . If a mechanic reverses a bad direction, the new direction . . . has its own dangers." Thus our EMDR expert, for example, has reversed her patient's terror and self-blame, but at the price of turning 1) the patient into a somewhat inflated source of ridicule and 2) turning herself into an all-good, all-powerful reverse mirror image of the mother: a relational role which cannot hold over time.

Paul Ornstein—the psychoanalyst/Holocaust survivor we spent the day with, a former collaborator of both Michael Balint and Heinz Kohut—was, like most thoughtful elders, more tolerant than I. All sorts of therapies have their place, he said, and he wasn't *a priori* offended by the language of "installing" and "uninstalling." "But you're right, the language people use does say something about what they're doing," he conceded.

His main concern was to make a distinction between technique-oriented therapy and process-oriented therapy, and he admitted that while he found EMDR interesting, he could never do it himself because "I won't interrupt a person's process. . . . I'm a purist." The details of his approach, following upon Kohut's own devotion to patients' subjective experience to the virtual exclusion of the therapist's authentic self, were no more congenial to me than EMDR. For my own part, I would feel hobbled and smothered if I didn't give myself the freedom to introduce my own reactions or even confront patients from time to time. The technique has to fit the therapist.

But in the end, theory and technique were not the point of listening to Paul Ornstein. The point was that he is the real thing, someone who has been through hell and not only survived to tell about it, but actually thrived without ever losing his immediate awareness of the inhumanity of which we humans are capable. His energy as he lectured made him appear, at certain moments, a much younger man; he modeled for us a vitality which refuses to repress any part of the whole truth of life, horrible or beautiful. Yet there was simplicity too, and a willingness to be baffled. I felt validated when this European intellectual, this eminent analyst who reads literature in several languages, concluded at one point: "Some people just stay hung up on the past!"

Ornstein told us that he had been an atheist even in his labor-camp days, an ethnic Jew only, but I could not help seeing him as a rabbi when he spoke of his group of young men mumbling prayers in the dark on Rosh Hashanna, holding hands and hoping their captors wouldn't hear. No, Ornstein is a rabbi after the heart of Martin Buber, who found God most completely in something that happens *between* people, and he has been religious in that sense all his life.

The day I returned home I happened "coincidentally" to hear from two older men that have been important psychotherapist-mentors for me, and that night I had the following dream:

I am a patient in a wheelchair that someone is pushing too fast, rolling quickly by a wall of tacked-up handbills such as one sees in Cambridge or Berkeley. One of the posters advertises a film that is a spoof on the Catholic priesthood. Clerics in robes are dancing comically. Whoever has been pushing me now turns into a mongrel dog which leaps up, trying to bite me over the back of the chair. I wake up swatting at it.

The religious reference has been changed to fit my own Roman Catholic ethnicity, but I think my unconscious is being pretty clear. Psychiatry is being rushed too fast and, far from learning the wisdom of its elders—its priesthood—it is mocking and dishonoring them. The mongrel dog—a chaotic and dangerous mix of good science, bad science, and market economics—needs to be evaded.

So please, reader, if you care, find one of these gems (most of them are not famous; there is probably one near you), these women and men who are our rabbis and our priests. Then, slow down and learn.

WHAT DOES SUFFERING DO?

"What is most important is what is most easily forgotten and can never be retold or retranslated enough." Here I retell the ancient story of wisdom-through-purification, which we see every day in the lives of those who survive prolonged and intense physical and emotional pain, with or without our help, and somehow emerge transformed. Psychotherapists do not make this happen, but, if they fail to bear witness to the process, an entire dimension of healing is lost. "Suffering" appeared in *Psychiatric Times*, October 2000.

An hour had passed in a sterile exam room at the VA Hospital. My disability evaluation was complete, thanks to honest and thoughtful answers from this Vietnam combat veteran, made with minimal eye contact. Feeling that I should give him something in return, I'd made a few informal suggestions about treatments that he might pursue. He didn't seem very interested.

Now he looked me in the face and delivered his evaluation. I was as glad for the utter self-possession he showed in making it as for the verdict itself. "You seem like an intelligent man," he said. "Have you ever read the *Psalms?*" And then this man, who lay awake nights alone in his trailer in northern Maine reading them, proceeded to recite from memory:

> *I am sinking in deep mire and there is no place to stand:*
> *I have come to deep waters and a flood overwhelms me.*
> *I have cried until I am exhausted.*
> *My days go up in smoke:*
> *My bones are inflamed as a bonfire.*

Like grass my heart is crushed and withered. . . .
I lie awake and feel like a sparrow alone on the roof.

—*Psalms* 69:2–3; 102:3–4,7; revised Berkeley version

"That David, he knew about pain," concluded the veteran.

It was the late 1980s. While junk-bond traders made millions, I had exhausted myself in the first few years of a minimally supervised private psychotherapy practice, trying (perhaps not unlike the bond traders) to "make things happen" for my roster of severely disturbed, often traumatized patients. Needing to regroup, I took a part-time job at the local VA doing psychiatric disability determinations. The idea was that no treatment would be involved. I took my time, walked over lunch and saw fewer patients than anyone else. The veterans often asked to see me again at the next required evaluation. I learned just how powerful listening alone can be, and I began to realize that there is a world of human suffering that forever dwarfs our puny interventions.

Just a few months ago, I sat discussing antidepressant medications with an orphaned, chronically depressed young woman in graduate school who was just beginning psychotherapy. Knuckling at her tears as she remembered her father, she asked with apprehension if medication would take these tears away. "At least this way I feel connected to myself," she said. From my time with the veterans (and many other experiences) I knew that in any intervention I might attempt with this woman, I would have to respect the fact that, like the psalmist, she valued her suffering.

Suffering. The word today has a largely archaic or technical usage, as in lawsuits alleging "pain and suffering" or medical case presentations in which patients "suffer from" something unearthed in the review of symptoms. Modern medicine (in the developed world) has given us options— some element of choice about when, where and how much we endure—and, of course, our primary response is one of thankfulness for the relief we now can, and should, provide for our patients. But then the need to name and consider suffering as a dimension of human experience may be, as it were, reduced to an icon on our busy screens.

If we want to understand the patients just described, and many others, we'd do well to click on it. We can't eliminate suffering, and some people still see suffering very differently than we do.

Many traditional religious approaches to suffering, as well as contemporary ones, both spiritual and scientific, center on a teleological discussion of what suffering is for. Such explanations have a natural appeal to desperate people looking for reasons why. If one "knows why" (or "what for"), there is some sense of control, even if the suffering can't be made to stop. I have speculated elsewhere that "knowing why"

169

for human beings serves the same protective function that "knowing when" they were next going to be shocked serves for those rats given a warning tone in learned helplessness experiments. (This group of animals does not develop the neuroendocrine abnormalities, characteristic of humans with posttraumatic stress disorder, that the unwarned animals do.)

For some suffering individuals, however, the immediate relief offered by causal or teleological explanations may turn into a tyrannical formula with which they can't possibly comply. In the days of the biblical Job, this formula was specifically religious: Do a better job obeying this or that law. Today we have dietary and exercise regimes of a secular nature; the diverse injunctions of self-help books; spiritual and pop-therapy leaders and movements; and, failing all else, psychiatry itself, either in its psychoanalytic version that claims to decode our histories and our symptoms, or in the pharmaceutical variety that purports to treat biological diseases. From Job facing his "comforters" to our patients facing us across our prescription pads, the common denominator is compliance.

And for Job, as for our patients, sometimes suffering just doesn't stop. The conclusions to draw are divergent: either the sufferer hasn't complied well enough yet (here is where treatment becomes tyrannical), or somebody's explanation is wrong (better said, incomplete).

Patients like either of the two above have been through many explanations and many treatments. If they seem, strangely enough, to value their suffering and to look upon the next facile answer with suspicion, we are well-advised to avoid seeing them as people who have lost hope. If they had, they wouldn't be here talking to us. The sleepless veteran reading the Psalms and the depressed young student finding a connection in her tears demonstrate a more profound and radical hope than ours, though they might not be able to express it. They choose to live as if their suffering were a transformative process.

Here is where the earthbound business that is clinical psychiatry has something to offer to philosophy, to ethics, to religion, to medicine itself. We who have known sufferers well over prolonged periods of time have seen some of them survive and come out the other side as changed people. We see their different patterns of relationship to self and others, their new attitudes toward life. Without having to believe in any religious or scientific theory, we know that suffering indeed can transform individuals and we can describe some of its results. We may not be in a position to answer the question, "What is suffering for?", but we can make as good a beginning as anyone in the direction of "What does suffering do?"

It would be difficult to round up such an outwardly diverse group for an outcome study, but any traditional psychiatrist (that is, any of us who have known patients well over periods of years) recognizes something special about certain people who emerge intact from a prolonged period of suffering. Whatever their history—physical or psychiatric illness, chronic intractable pain, catastrophic loss, sexual abuse, prison camps—these inspiring individuals have an unshakable acceptance of self that does not submit to the judgments of others. They don't compare themselves with or compete with anyone. They make themselves heard, but don't try to impose a personal agenda on others, and, more than leading their lives, they are open to going where life leads them. Compassionate and receptive, they tend to be rooted in the present moment, all in one place rather than conflicted and at war with themselves. Regardless of overt religious beliefs, or lack of them, they embody the connectedness to other people and the living world that many of our greatest religious teachers have held as a penultimate value.

How did these people get this way? Apart from shutting down the production of brain-derived neurotropic protein in our hippocampi (as it undoubtedly does), what does suffering do?

In fact, this transformative process has been well-described, from the inside, by those who have lived through or witnessed it. These accounts, almost as old as the written word itself, range from the ancient Hebrew poetry with which this essay began (most famously, in the book of *Job*), through Juan de la Cruz's *Dark Night of the Soul* in the 16th century, down to the writings of poets, novelists and depth psychologists in our own day (one of my own modern favorites is Kat Duff's *The Alchemy of Illness*). With those above two patients in mind, I will re-trace this perennial description here on the theory that what is most important is what is most easily forgotten and can never be retold or re-translated enough.

The most fundamental lesson sufferers learn flows directly from the failure of explanation: No one is in control. Typically, they begin by struggling to comply with a preconceived treatment process or regime that promises deliverance in accordance with some explanation of their plight. Whether the effort goes into tolerating the side effects of a mood stabilizer, sitting for hours in meditation practice, or bringing the "right" dreams or insights to the analyst, someone else's idea of what the sufferer needs is not the hoped-for answer. Thus failing behaviorally, the sufferer may yet seek solace in an imagined past or future constructed from the governing explanation: "If only I had . . ." or "I'll feel better when . . ."

When this tack yields at last to rage and/or despair, when it becomes clear that being a good boy or girl doesn't work and that Authority is not in control, the first hidden fruit of the suffering process starts to blossom in the dark. This is autonomy, an acceptance of one's own perceptions and needs as valid apart from externally derived values, judgments and comparisons.

Blake, William (1737–1827). "Job's Evil Dreams." Illustrations of the Book of Job, III,45, pl.11. Watercolor. Copyright The Pierpont Morgan Library; Art Resource, NY.

Now that ego—or Will —is on its own, internal judgment replaces external compliance in the person's attempt to get control of the suffering. Contemporary psychiatry sees this as entirely pathological: "excessive or inappropriate guilt" (cf. item 2 on the Hamilton Depression Rating Scale and items 5 and 6 on the Beck Inventory).

This psychiatric attitude may be taken with compassion as well as objectivity, but it closes off any further understanding of suffering as a process. Some patients feel distanced or even abandoned by such medical-model reassurance. This was certainly true of the graduate student described above, for whom inexplicable guilt was a dominant theme.

In other ages and cultures there were helpful vocabularies available to sufferers like this young woman: well-described sins to atone for (Christianity) or earthly attachments from which to free oneself (Buddhism). The "searching and fearless moral inventory" of Bill W's Fourth Step in Alcoholics Anonymous is one contemporary replacement for these. This patient is not looking for reassurance, but for my help in inventing a vocabulary of her own. And, as good a person as she already is, she will no doubt become a better one by following this moral imperative for quite some distance.

As the suffering process wears on, though, the internal judge becomes every bit as tyrannical as any external authority. William Blake captures this well in a painting of Job's tortured dreaming. The figure that persecutes him is identical to himself, except for the Devil's cloven hoof in lieu of a left foot. Boiling in his own juices, the sufferer finds that even the fiercest self-examination will not make the suffering stop. He is not in control, either. Sooner or later, these agonies free the ego from its oppressive dream of finally getting it right. Finally, there is nothing left for the sufferer to do but defy all judges internal and external; accept, forgive and love himself; and then face whatever happens.

Jung once described our job as helping patients to "hang on until nature grants a reprieve." That reprieve is more often a quiet and gradual miracle than a dramatic turn like Job's vision of God in the whirlwind. But when it comes—and it can come even to the dying and to the chronically ill and disabled—it is experienced as a gift, only secondarily connected to anything the sufferer or his allies (including us) may have done.

Perhaps ill or scarred, certainly imperfect and fallible, the survivor of suffering emerges still somehow more vital, more intact as a human self than many who have never lost soundness of mind or body. All of us can think of great figures from history and literature who fit this description: an Abraham Lincoln or a William Blake come to mind. More importantly, most psychiatrists can point to these same attributes among our patients, though such individuals may be less articulate, or known only to a family or a neighborhood.

In human history, many more sufferers have fallen off the road I have briefly described than followed the process through to this idealized end. Some have been destroyed literally; others psychically, ending in resignation, embitterment, addiction. Now medical science, including ours in psychiatry, can help many more to "hang on." What kind of world is this going to make?

If we doctors have no awareness of the transformative process that suffering engenders in some of our patients, if we simply abort or arrest suffering whenever possible with our technologies before listening for the meanings our patients may find in it, we may unwittingly contribute to a society flattened of emotional depth, a compassionless culture that retreats behind locked gates from the less fortunate.

But if we listen with respect to patients like the ones I have described, who are trying to survive rather than avoid this mysterious process they have discerned within themselves, then the world may yet become a better place—and we will have helped.

PSYCHOTHERAPY AFTER MOHAMMED ATTA

I spent September 11, 2001 shuttling back and forth between therapy sessions and a friend's apartment across the alley where the television played and replayed terrorist Mohammed Atta's millennial Dance of Death; he had flown out of Portland earlier that morning. In the days that followed I was surprised to find that my work did not seem reduced to utter insignificance. In fact, I felt an added urgency—not to speed things up for people, but to try harder to connect with whatever was alive in my patients, even if that vitality constellated around such "mundane" therapeutic issues as marital discord, conflicts with a boss, a feeling of not being recognized for one's value, and the like. There was a heightened sense of energy and purpose that, in the main, has lasted. I was reminded of William Saroyan's adage, "In the time of your life, live!"

I tried, in this piece (_Psychiatric Times_, February 2002), to put a larger historical and archetypal context around my continued, and renewed, identity as a psychotherapist.

Portland, Maine can now lay claim to another famous man. Like our poet Longfellow, he was inclined to champion those dispossessed from ancestral homelands. And like Joshua Chamberlain, the theologian/general who won the battle of Gettysburg, he was an imaginative tactician with a fondness for scripture. He shopped in our Walmart, ate at our Pizza Hut, and slept at our Comfort Inn. His name was Mohammed Atta.

The stylish Atta was first spotted here by an observer I consider reliable in late August, in the company of some regular Arabic-speaking customers at a local convenience store. Beyond that report, Atta sightings have multiplied, as always happens in the nascent phases of a myth.

175

Waitresses are sure they served him, librarians that he used our Public Library's computers several times. But the Egyptian lawyer's son had long before succumbed to the temptation of becoming something more (or less) than human. In methodically orchestrating the deadliest terrorist attack in American history, he became the latest incarnation of an archetype: the Devil to us, and (since the archetypal world is always and ever polarized) the great Martyred Hero to others. Jung's term for Mohammed Atta's fate was "identification with the collective psyche." In its grip, one becomes "the fortunate possessor of *the* great truth," manifesting "megalomania in the . . . familiar form it takes in the reformer, the prophet, and the martyr." Jung had good reason to emphasize this particular pathology, having been himself taken in by it for a time in the guise of Adolf Hitler.

While January 1st, 2001 officially began the new millennium, September 11th was our millennial event. The devil-hero Atta, like Hitler before him, embodies the "Rough Beast" that Yeats foretold, the one that "slouches toward Bethlehem to be born." Like the final, sudden crack of an earthquake, September 11th was the result of powerful and unseen forces—in this case, cultural forces—whose shifting has been underway for many decades. These forces have been pushing what we psychiatrists sometimes call the human Self away from historically recent developments in the direction of individuality, and back toward more typical, collective forms.

The Self, as we and our patients experience it, is not an immutable aspect of human nature whose basic form we can take for granted. In many important aspects this Self is a culturally determined phenomenon, and it has been changing fast even during the brief time that psychodynamic psychiatrists have been around to describe it. And today, whether 21st century humans memorize the Koran or wear Tommy Hilfiger jeans, they are increasingly defined by what they belong to and not what they uniquely and individually are. We are being subsumed into a world of collective symbols. It is fitting that Mohammed Atta ate his last meal at Pizza Hut before he steered a jumbo jet into the World Trade Center. His world and ours is a world of brand names.

Some of us had seen this new cultural context coming, but we are all, finally, surprised by it. Barely a century old, the tradition of psychodynamic psychotherapy—by which I mean here, those therapies whose aim is to restore and develop the Self rather than only to modify behaviors—now finds itself pivotally placed. Therapists occupy this position not only because of our various skills in treating anxiety and psychological trauma. Most fundamentally, we find ourselves here because we advocate for the healing potential of individuation. In doing so, we offer an alternative both to the rantings of bin Laden and to the videos of Britney Spears.

We may debate whether or not the pursuit of uniqueness in helping individual patients to understand the themes and plots of their own lives has any ultimate value. We may even persuasively argue that the pursuit of uniqueness actually further alienates our patients from an increasingly collective world, leading them away from the comforts of fitting in. But we can't deny the fact that this pursuit is the foundation of our profession. Psychodynamic psychotherapy stands in opposition to the individual's imprisonment by any set of collective symbols which would wholly define his or her identity. Whether they are a response to material deprivation (radical Islam) or to toxic overabundance (MTV), we have learned that collective symbols, taken literally, impoverish the soul.

Writing in New York before the Trade Towers fell, the historian Jacques Barzun described in detail the course of a 500-year experiment in Western culture which was coming to a close as he worked. This experiment had involved the development of individual selves on an unprecedented, mass scale. Its inaugural event, the one whose opposite bookend would prove to be the September 11 disaster, was Martin Luther's challenge to the Catholic hierarchy, 95 propositions nailed to the church door in Wittenberg in 1517 which questioned the Church's right to determine the status of the individual before God. Luther's was a civilized kind of "attack" on another building which stood for the reigning power structure.

In medieval Europe until then, collectively defined human selves had found their identities as part of something. Peasantry, clergy, noblemen all found their place in a putatively "divine" social scheme. An elite priesthood, literate in Latin, communicated the conventional behavioral prescriptions by means of images and icons, whose penultimate form was the didactic stained-glass window. These prescriptions included explanations of, and acceptable channels for, the various unruly human passions. For the most part, the illiterate masses complied, faithfully fulfilling their pre-ordained duties. The only alternative in their society was to be marginalized. But Luther's "attack" was emblematic—like the earthquake's final crack—of a cultural shift that had long been in process. Printing presses, literacy in vernacular languages, geographical mobility, the growth of the money economy: all these conspired to give more and more opportunity to the autonomous, self-defining, questioning individual.

This historical process gathered momentum. By the nineteenth and twentieth centuries in the West, vast numbers of adults were reading novels, poetry, history, science; they looked within themselves and recorded private reflections; they developed critical perspectives on their own societies; they sought personal meaning in their lives and engaged in the "pursuit of happiness." Apart from tiny, privileged minorities earlier in human history (Socrates' Athenian friends, Molière's court audiences), all of this was new. Psychotherapy, a child of the twentieth century, brought the verbal, dialogic search for truth, beauty and the well-lived life out of the books and to the wide public in an immediate, interactive way. Scientific reasoning, philosophical ideas, and the narrative constructions of literature were all brought to bear on the lives and problems of ordinary people in the consulting room.

Although it was defined within society as a purchasable medical service, psychotherapy nevertheless encouraged patients to develop, from their emotional distress or their psychiatric symptoms, a critique of the social structures within which they, the patients, were embedded. And when this evolving insight went any further afield than the patient's family of origin, it was potentially subversive. And further afield it must go, for as Karen Horney recognized at the outset, our patients experience "the culturally determined difficulties in an accentuated form, mostly through the medium of childhood experiences."

The hidden radicalism of traditional forms of psychotherapy lay in their attempt to cure by the development of awareness of social contexts, and thus freeing patients from the self-defining influence of those contexts. Jung called this attempt one at "wakening from the collective dream." Whether by untangling therapeutic transference, by reexamining the family of origin, or by looking at conflictual aspects of everyday life in the present, patients healed themselves by becoming different, unique. More than just wholly unconscious products of social influences, patients in therapy became independent selves able to reflect on those influences. Thus, in retrospect, psychotherapy can be seen as a final, democratic flowering of the Western experiment in individualism.

This idealized account belies the fact that it was ending even as it began. The same conditions which allowed psychotherapy to briefly flourish also incubated a powerful new influence toward conformity: the neofeudal culture of the corporation, which in all but name replaced the nation-state as the dominant form of social organization by the late 20th century. Psychiatrists, whose working conditions are now structured by the corporate culture—whether they practice in hospitals, clinics or private practices—are entirely familiar with its constraints. Psychotherapy's subversive potential has been eviscerated by this culture, leaving short-term and medication-based approaches as the whole of mainstream mental health care. These approaches' avowed aim is the adaptation of the individual to the social status quo.

Some critics (notably the psychoanalyst Philip Cushman) even argue that much of the "high-end" traditional therapy that remains available functions as an unwitting accomplice of corporate culture. With its boutique-like focus on an ever-unsatisfied self and its personal needs, a socially naive psychodynamic therapy may simply encourage patients to be good consumers.

But corporate culture has a more direct servant, whose evolution closely paralleled that of psychotherapy in the last century. Like psychotherapy, it too promised happiness. This was commercial advertising. Its genius lay in harnessing the individualistic impulse toward limitless choice, and channeling it into collective forms of expression. These purchasable joys—be they a mouthwash, a timeshare on some tropical beach, or the newest anxiolytic—are sold for their purported transformative or "therapeutic" results. Cushman ironically captures this in quoting an advertisement: "Thirty-nine flavors. Find yourself."

And so, long before September 11th, 2001, Western culture was already well on its way toward a new, secular medievalism. In this digital-electronic age our new icons are not stained-glass windows but TV commercials, corporate logos, clinical algorithms reproduced on Power-Point slides. Our saints are TV and film celebrities, pop music stars, professional athletes (not the people themselves, but the images crafted for and superimposed upon them). Our secular priesthood's arcane literacy is not in Church Latin, but in what Jacques Barzun calls "techne": the sciences which promise control of how information is transduced, be they computer programming, genetic engineering, marketing psychology—or psychopharmacology.

Thus, it makes perfect sense that the modern West finds among its final archenemies the radicalized wing of a resurgent religion which was born in the original Middle Ages, and which only fifty years ago was thought by scholars to be an antiquated and dying faith. The Crusades metaphor, offered inadvertently by President Bush and seized upon by the Taliban and its allies, is more accurate than we would like to think. But now the West marches under the brand-name banners of globalization, not the cross.

The potential role of psychotherapy in this polarized social context is best introduced by a poignant anecdote. A Washington, D.C. colleague of mine happened to have his car in the shop during the time of the September attacks and, depending on taxis to get around, found himself riding to work with a bearded Afghani driver. The driver had hung Rosary beads from the mirror and an American flag from the turn-signal rod, as if these symbols could counteract the sudden symbolism of his own appearance. Together they listened to the ongoing radio news. At the end of his ride, my friend asked the driver, "How's it going . . . you know, with the Rosary beads and the flag?" The driver replied quietly, "Pretty good so far."

The connection these two men had was made possible by my colleague's spontaneous act of psychotherapy. Both became aware, as individuals, of their mutual victimization by the black-and-white tyranny of collective symbols. Each saw the other as a vulnerable human being.

For an instant they became a conscious community of two selves: I and Thou commiserating over the idling of a taxicab.

Around them, the Rough Beast slouches forward; the human psyche stands poised to enter another cycle of possession by archetypal dominants. The very possibility of conscious, reflective community, which our fledgling tradition has helped to create, offers a flickering hope. We psychotherapists are among those whose job it will be to guard and carry forward that hope.

THE DOMESTICATION
OF THE TRUTH

In *Let Us Now Praise Famous Men*, James Agee wrote that "every fury on earth has been absorbed in time. . . . Official acceptance is the one unmistakable symptom that salvation has been beaten again." Absorption, normalization, assimilation; the radical message sinks to the bottom of the pond and the ripples eventually die out. Here, in one individual's therapy, I called this process "domestication."

True physicians (regardless of credentialed discipline) are distinguished by an awareness that some wounds should not be allowed to heal too soon, that to heal from the bottom, these must be kept open.

"Truth" appeared in *Psychiatric Times* in February 2001.

The patient, an overworked, middle-aged primary care physician, has more than once told me what led him to his choice of career. Misunderstood by his father, poised between the culture of the "old country" and that of the urban United States, he had found a unique comfort, as a boy, sitting in the big leather armchair of his own family's physician and chatting with him. This general feeling, more than anything scientific, was what he had hoped to provide for his own patients. We often commiserate about the social forces and bureaucratic systems that have conspired to keep us both from regularly and easily reaching this goal that we have in common.

My patient's commitments will not allow a wholesale changing of horses in midstream. His temperament might be better suited to the writing of poetry (which he used to love), but he will have to play out his medical career a good while longer. Yet, an incomplete response to psychotherapy and medication for his syndrome of anxious depression has convinced me that some concession to the needs of his own nature must be made, and I, in turn, have been trying to convince him of this.

While this is easy enough on an intellectual level, the psychophysiological mandate of the introspective poet is soon translated into the problem-solving idiom of the physician. Don't book appointments after 3 p.m. on Thursdays. Take a yoga class. Walk to work.

But Thursday afternoons fill up with dictations, paperwork, phone calls; yoga class conflicts with the kids' soccer games; he needs to take the car for hospital rounds. Both of us see what is happening, but it happens all the same.

One day, after another attempted cutback in work hours, he brings in a dream. A mute, "slapstick" version of himself is tied by the wrists ("poseyed," in medical slang) to a chair, but keeps getting loose and coming after him in a half-comical, half-menacing kind of way. My patient can't tell if the slapstick man wants to play or wants to hurt him. With difficulty, non-verbal persuasion and duct tape (that most universal of solutions) my patient gets his alter self back into the chair. But then the slapstick man gets loose again! And so on.

The truth of a person (definition postponed) is a wild creature. It cannot be domesticated or indefinitely restrained. Micromanagement of the office schedule and time at the gym will not keep the slapstick man chair-bound. This dream figure has gotten across to the doctor in a way that I could not, and we are now in agreement: Our job is to find out what this mute fellow really wants.

I underline the point with some imagery from just outside my window. In our coastal city there is the frequent summertime sight of sea kayaks on the roofs of cars. Whoever rents the parking spot below appears to install his or her kayak atop the Volvo in May and remove it in October, as if to be ever-ready for the spontaneous whim to throw the boat into the harbor and paddle away. But I monitor the spot: The Volvo-kayak is always there when I come in and still there when I leave. While I may hope otherwise, I suspect that the boat's primary function is to proclaim to the world that its owner has a soul (and perhaps to remind the owner as well).

We do this, all of us; we throw bones to the truth and try to keep it tied down. It wants to play freely in our lives, but its full implications threaten us. This is as true of cultures as it is of individuals. I think of the gospels layering Pauline theology over the words of Jesus, or later, of analytic institutes freeze-drying the insights of Freud and Jung. I think of the tired 12-bar blues played in bars coast to coast; buried beneath it, the tortured freestyle cries of Robert Johnson. We can't seem to bear the truth for very long. The weight of cultural accretions "takes down" the truth like a wrestler.

What do I mean here by truth, as an attribute of a person? Simply the expression of one's own essential being: whether actively, by doing or receptively, by seeing. But in either case, doing or seeing in the way that the individual uniquely does or sees. Some theologians place us here as the eyes with which God sees his creation, or the hands with which he furthers it. I haven't come up with a more scientifically correct way to put it. We may envy the conventionally religious, for whom the question "What was I put on this earth to do?" has an unequivocally clarifying effect. But whether we personally prefer to believe that some purpose already exists for each of us to find or that we only make one up for ourselves out of the raw materials of our lives, our task remains the same. Our beliefs are irrelevant to the psychological imperative embodied by the relentlessly approaching slapstick man.

In the physician's case, truth led, not to rest and relaxation, but to more work (as it often does). This work connected the introverted poet with a new and surprisingly outer-directed passion that would affect many lives. But the poet's eye remained and also found solace in a decidedly non-New Age pastime: tying flies under the tutelage of an older man who liked and appreciated him just as the doctor with the leather armchair had, many years before.

THE OWL STICK

I close this section, and this second edition of my book, with a reminiscence from two decades' distance, published in *a Voices* issue
on the theme of "Rituals in Psychotherapy: Beginnings and
Endings" (Winter 2001). It was not intended as an example of
good therapy, adequate management of the transference, or any
other such thing. I tried instead to be as honest as I could about
the hazards and rewards of learning to be my own kind of therapist, and my bewilderment on finding that I have somehow
halfway succeeded.

From a certain distance we smile at the youthful fiction that our techniques and our boundaries can protect us from a plain fact: we therapists,
like our patients, are forever falling apart and pulling ourselves back
together. The firm ground we try to supply for them actually cracks and
shifts beneath our own feet.

We smile, even as we substitute for technique wise-sounding myths
with happy endings which explain, in retrospect, what "really" went on and
how we happen still to be here with our shingles still hung and patients
still coming in. Trying to ignore, at this little distance, the plain truth that
the ground still moves and we persist only by the grace of God.

At this distance our therapy is as scattered as any nocturnal dream.
I was 31, immature, beginning to fall apart. She tried to look all grown
up at 21 and had never been put together. Cassette players blasting, we
drove long rural distances from opposite directions to meet in a dim,
sublet office. Her father had done a lot of damage, but my hearing about
it did nothing much; the attractions of alcohol, drugs, and "acting
out"—better said, avenging herself—were far too powerful. I was failing to help her, failing to protect her. But we were both musicians, and
we would swap tapes of various favorite performers, introducing each
other to our own heroes and our own solaces.

184

It was a time of trying on identities; without them, or in between them, we walked raw in the world. I recall one day this classically preppie-looking young woman arriving in a black cut-off motorcycle T-shirt with a picture of a Viking ship on it. "Harley-Davidson: The Spirit of Adventure," it read. I sat meanwhile drinking hot water with honey, afraid for my health. "Guzzling coffee again?" she inquired, and howled with laughter when I told her what was in the mug.

Another time, crying —I think it was her father again—she reached for the tissue and found I had bought the store brand. This was before cheap computer graphics, so generics came in a plain brown box. "Paul! Generic tissue! *Generic* tissue!?" She laughed through her tears, but her point was apt. I was overwhelmed by my practice and the store brand emphatically said so, said that I could only give the minimum. (I have since raised my minimum to Kleenex brand, with the flowers on it.)

I remember my own process much better than hers. Wandering in the woods before a session, I would hope for a reprieve from being sucked down into the Whirlpool and look for it in the ripe rotten smell of leaves in late fall, pink glimpses of lady's-slippers in spring. Trapped in the endings of things, one is given a vivid awareness of other things beginning. Such things may not save us, but they are there, and are all that we have. These sights and sounds and smells would be my supplies, my sustenance for going further down and deeper in.

Towards the end of our three years together she brought me what seemed to be a dream of her birth. She was being dragged behind a pickup truck at high speed with chains or ropes, through and then out of a muddy, weed-choked lake. The dream corresponded to the details of her mother's precipitous labor, but I see now that it also described what was happening to each of us at that very time.

Finally she opted for the geographic cure. Her parents had long since stopped paying, so she left owing me a sizeable balance. Considering the shape she was in by that time, this almost felt fair to me, but she promised to pay when she could.

In our last session I was moved to read her a certain Cree poem (in Howard Norman's translation). I read the poem while ending work with a few other people to whom I had felt particularly connected to during that time, but I never thought of this reading as any kind of ritual until now.

With you I want to carve
the owl stick.
With your help
we'll carve it.

The crow stick failed.
So what.

The duck stick failed.
So what.

This is different.
This time.

They'll see it fly, owl.
They'll hear it call, owl.
They'll say "Owl stick lives nearby."

And they'll stop gossiping
about those two old ones
always carving, night and day.

A month or so later she called from another state. She'd met a man at a bar, he'd had some heroin, and now she'd woken up alone on an apartment floor. Feeling only more defeated, I advised her to sign herself in to a residential drug rehab facility. This wasn't what she wanted to hear, and she hung up.

Next, for a couple of years, I got (and then sent) Christmas cards. Somehow she had righted herself, gotten a good job, started college. In her final letter to me she enclosed a check for what she had left owing, several thousand dollars. She wrote that she still often remembered things I had said to her in our therapy together. I don't remember a single thing I said, only some of her own aphoristic statements, which had seemed to emerge from some wise crone within this confused young woman. That, and the dangerous theatricality of her acting out, some of which approached performance art in its inventiveness.

What I keep from our time together, apart from the fragments here described, is the conviction that she and I were more than just haphazard mirrors for one another. There was a mutual appreciation of real things belonging to the other, and often, a willingness to learn from and respond to each other that operates more freely in people as yet "unformed." Elusive and ephemeral as they were to ourselves, our strong parts did recognize and make contact with each other, which strengthened both of us for the road ahead.

• • • • •

Reading the above with a friend a few days later, I have to agree that there is a quality here of romance remembered (although romance in the literal sense never happened). Perhaps the best I could do for this patient at the time was cross her boundaries, and let her cross mine, in a less damaging way than her father had done. Sometimes I wonder whether any of us can ever do better than that; whether *any* useful therapy happens without a crossing of boundaries. I doubt it. But I try now at least to be more conscious of such crossings, and to label them explicitly at times, thus sharing the responsibility with patients.

To go further into life, this young woman did well to get away from me. I had given her what I could. The entire underlying pattern of blurred boundaries, of too much wide-open intimacy with a man, had to go. Apparently it got worse before it got better, played out to its logical conclusion, and then, one hopes, a more autonomous intimacy became possible. But I was part of the geography this woman needed to cure herself of. And that, I think, is as much why she paid me as anything helpful I might have said. The debt was a lingering connection. She payed it, like a real grown-up.

To my friend I will admit to the romantic longing in this reminiscence, less for the patient as a person (much as I liked her) than for those days when we were innocents together, as in the old song:

Well, we ain't got a barrel o' money
Maybe we're ragged and funny
But we'll travel along
Singin' a song
Side by side.

You don't survive this long as a therapist unless Innocence learns from Experience, Romance is tempered by Tragedy and near-tragedy. Maybe that is how God's grace works. The hard trick is to keep Innocence and its healing power alive even as we learn how vulnerable it makes us; to protect ourselves and yet remain open to the Other at the same time. If you have found out how to do this, let me know. I'm still carving, night and day.

REFERENCE NOTES

Part I

"Dream Rebuts Therapist"

Bollas, C. (1987). Normotic Illness. *The Shadow of the Object*, pp.135-156. London: Free Association Books.

Gabel, S. (1993). The phenomenology of the self and its objects in waking and dreaming: Implications for a model of dreaming. *Journal of the American Academy of Psychoanalysis* 21(3):339-362.

Gloor, P., et.al. (1982). The role of the limbic system in experiential phenomena of temporal lobe epilepsy. *Annals of Neurology* 12(2):129-142.

Hillman, J. (1979). *The Dream and the Underworld*. New York: Harper & Row.

Klerman, G., et. al. (1994). *Interpersonal Therapy of Depression*. Northvale, NJ: Aronson.

"Catfish on the Bottom"

Jung, C.G. (1966). Fundamental principles in the treatment of collective identity. *The Collected Works of Carl G. Jung, vol.7: Two Essays on Analytical Psychology*, ed. W. McGuire, pp. 288-300. Princeton: Bollingen.

Winnicott, D.W.(1989). Nothing at the centre. *Psycho-Analytic Explorations*, pp. 49-52. Cambridge MA: Harvard.

"The Permanent Trip"

Abraham, H.D. (1983). Visual phenomenology of the LSD flashback. *Archives of General Psychiatry* 40:884-88.

American Psychiatric Association (1994). *Diagnostic and Statistical Manual of Mental Disorders*, Fourth Edition (DSM-IV). Washington DC: American Psychiatric Association.

"Lacan at Bonus Bagels"

Lacan, J. (1977). The mirror stage. *Ecrits: A Selection*, pp. 1-7. New York: W.W. Norton.

"Living with Doubt"

Genova, P. (1993). Reality by decree: A transference hazard in the therapy of the sexually abused. *Psychiatric Times* 10(11), November 1993.

Kluft, R. (1989). Playing for time: Temporizing techniques in the treatment of Multiple Personality Disorder. *American Journal of Clinical Hypnosis* 32(2): 90-98.

Putnam, F. (1989). *Diagnosis and Treatment of Multiple Personality Disorder.* New York: Guilford.

"The New Covenant"

American Psychiatric Association (1993). Practice guideline for major depressive disorder in adults. *American Journal of Psychiatry* 150 (4), supplement.

Beck, A.T. (1976). *Cognitive Therapy and the Emotional Disorders.* New York: International Universities Press.

Bollas, C. (1993). Unconscious communication: Wakeful dreaming in psychotherapy. Presentation at the Institute and Conference of the American Academy of Psychotherapists, Santa Fe, NM, November 1993.

Butler, S.F. & Strupp, H.H. (1986). Specific and nonspecific factors in psychotherapy: A problematic paradigm for psychotherapy research. *Psychotherapy* 23:30-40.

Erickson, M.H. (1980). *The Collected Papers of Milton H. Erickson on Hypnosis, vol. 4. Innovative Hypnotherapy*, ed. E. L. Rossi. New York: Irvington.

Freud, S. (1914/1953). The Moses of Michelangelo. *The Standard Edition of the Complete Psychological Works of Sigmund Freud*, vol. 13, ed. J. Strachey, pp. 209-238. London: Hogarth Press.

Jung, C.G. (1952/1960). Synchronicity: An acausal connecting principle. *The Collected Works of Carl G. Jung*, vol. 8, ed. W. McGuire, pp. 417-519. Princeton: Bollingen.

Jung, C.G. (1961). *Memories, Dreams, Reflections.* New York: Random House.

Kohut, H. (1971). *The Restoration of the Self.* New York: International Universities Press.

Winnicott, D.W. (1965). *The Maturational Processes and the Facilitating Environment.* New York: International Universities Press.

189

"'I'm Not Your Urban Renewal Project'"

Buber, M. (1970). *I and Thou*. New York: Scribner's.

Habermas, J. (1992). *Postmetaphysical Thinking*. Cambridge, MA: MIT Press.

Harlow, H. (1958). The nature of love. *American Psychologist* 133: 677-

Kojève, A. (1969). *Introduction to the Reading of Hegel*. New York: Basic Books.

Krishnamurti, J. (1973) *The Awakening of Intelligence*. New York: Harper & Row.

van der Kolk et.al. (1996). *Traumatic Stress*. New York: Guilford.

Part II

"The Thaw"

Kernberg, O. (1984). *Severe Personality Disorders*. New Haven CT: Yale.

Kohut, H. (1971). *The Restoration of the Self*. New York: International Universities Press.

"Snow White"

Grimm, J., and Grimm, W.(1987). Snow White. In Zipes, J. (trans.), *The Complete Fairy Tales of the Brothers Grimm*. New York: Ballantine Books.

Gruen, A. (1988). *The Betrayal of the Self*. New York: Grove Press.

Hillman, J. (1975). Betrayal. *Loose Ends: Primary Papers in Archetypal Psychology*, pp. 63-81. Dallas, TX: Spring Books.

Pinker, S. (1997). *How the Mind Works*. New York: W.W. Norton.

"Raffaela's Hug"

Wright, R. (1994). *The Moral Animal*. New York: Random House.

"'I Just Keep Playing the Same Note'"

Krishnamurti, J. (1973) *The Awakening of Intelligence*. New York: Harper & Row.

"Getting Two (2.0) People into the Room"

Kohut, H. (1971). *The Restoration of the Self*. New York: International Universities Press.

Winnicott, D.W. (1989). The importance of the setting in meeting regression in psychoanalysis. *Psycho-Analytic Explorations*, pp.96-102. Cambridge, MA: Harvard.

"The Endless Walk of the Fool"

Hillman, J. (1975). Pothos: The nostalgia of the Puer Eternus. *Loose Ends*, pp. 49-62. Dallas TX: Spring Publications.

"Rockabye Baby: Winnicott's Hatred"

Little, M. (1990) *Psychotic Anxieties and Containment: A Personal Record of an Analysis with Winnicott.* Northvale NJ: Aronson.

Winnicott, D.W. (1957). Hate in the countertransference. *Collected Papers: Through Paediatrics to Psychoanalysis.* New York: Basic Books.

"Our Trainees' Calling, Our Job Description"

Cushman, P. (1995). *Constructing the Self, Constructing America: A Cultural History of Psychotherapy.* Reading MA: Addison-Wesley.

Gustafson, J.P. (1995). *Brief versus Long Psychotherapy.* Northvale NJ: Aronson.

Gustafson, J.P. (1995). *The Dilemmas of Brief Therapy.* New York: Plenum.

Hillman, J. (1979). Peaks and vales: The soul/spirit distinction as basis for the differences between psychotherapy and spiritual discipline. *Puer Papers*, ed. J.Hillman, pp.54-74. Dallas TX: Spring Publications.

Miller, A. (1981). *Prisoners of Childhood.* New York: Basic Books.

Trungpa, C. (1987). *Cutting Through Spiritual Materialism.* Boston: Shambhala Publications.

Part III

"God or Vending Machine"

American Psychiatric Association (1994). *Diagnostic and Statistical Manual of Mental Disorders,* Fourth Edition (DSM-IV). Washington DC: American Psychiatric Association.

Kramer, P. (1993). *Listening to Prozac.* New York: Viking.

"Requiem for Psychoanalysis"

Eigen, M. (1992). *Coming through the Whirlwind.* Wilmette IL: Chiron Publications.

Gustafson, J. (1995). *Brief versus Long Psychotherapy.* Northvale NJ: Aronson.

Linehan, M. (1993). *Cognitive-Behavioral Treatment of Borderline Personality Disorder.* New York: Guilford.

Stern, D. (1985). *The Interpersonal World of the Infant.* New York: Basic Books.

"The Shifting Metaphors of Biological Psychiatry"

Critser, G. (1996). Oh, how happy we will be! Pills, paradise, and the profits of the drug companies. *Harper's Magazine*, June 1996, pp. 39-48.

Diller, L. (1996). The run on Ritalin: Attention Deficit Disorder and stimulant treatment in the 1990's. *Hastings Center Report* 26(2):12-18.

Fancher, R. (1995). Biological psychiatry's confusion of tongues. In Fancher, *Cultures of Healing*. New York: Freeman.

Gustafson, J. (unpublished). The John Wayne myth and the bipolar dilemma.

"The Coming Polarization of Psychotherapy"

American Psychiatric Association (1994). *Diagnostic and Statistical Manual of Mental Disorders, Fourth Edition* (DSM-IV). Washington DC: American Psychiatric Association.

Buber, M. (1970) *I and Thou*. New York: Scribner's.

Jacques, E.(1970). Death and the mid-life crisis. *Work, Creativity and Social Justice*. London: Heinemann.

Jung, C.G. (1968). Commentary on *The Secret of the Golden Flower. The Collected Works of Carl G. Jung*, vol. 13: Alchemical Studies, ed. W. McGuire. Princeton: Bollingen.

Kramer, P. (1993) *Listening to Prozac*. New York: Viking.

Seligman, M. (1974). Depression and learned helplessness. *The Psychology of Depression*, ed. R. Friedman and M. Katz. Washington, DC: Winston.

Tolstoy, L. (1981). *The Death of Ivan Illyich*. New York: Bantam.

Troyat, H. (1980). *Tolstoy*. New York: Harmony.

Winnicott, D.W. (1989). Fear of breakdown. *Psycho-Analytical Explorations*, pp.87-95. Cambridge, MA: Harvard.

"Psychiatric Wisdom"

Bellah, R., et.al. (1985). *Habits of the Heart*. Berkeley: University of California.

Genova, P. (1993). A good goodbye: Is American psychiatry terminally ill? *Psychiatric Times* 10(6), June 1993.

Hillman, J. (1975). A note on story. *Loose Ends*, pp.1-4. Dallas, TX: Spring Publications.

Langs, R. (1985). *Madness and Cure*. Emerson NJ: Newconcept Press.

Part IV

"Is American Psychiatry Terminally Ill?"

Luhrmann, T. (2001). *Of Two Minds*. New York: Vintage.
McNamara, M. (1994). *Breakdown*. New York: Pocket Books.
Rako, S. and Mazer, H., eds. (1983). *Semrad: The Heart of a Therapist*. Northvale, NJ: Jason Aronson.

"Boundary Violations and the Fall from Eden"

Brown, J. et al. (1996). A defect in nurturing in mice lacking the immediate early gene *fosB*. *Cell* 86: 297–309.
Fodor, J. (1998). The trouble with psychological Darwinism. *London Review of Books*, 22 January 1998, 11–13.
Wright, R. (1994). *The Moral Animal*. New York: Random House.

"There Are Really Only Three Kinds of Psychotherapy"

Buber, M. (1970). *I and Thou*. New York: Scribner's.
Habermas, J. (1992). *Postmetaphysical Thinking*. Cambridge MA: MIT Press.
Linehan, M. (1993). *Cognitive-Behavioral Therapy of Borderline Personality Disorder*. New York: Guilford.
Winnicott, D.W. (1989) On "The Use of an Object." *Psycho-Analytic Explorations*, 217–239. Cambridge MA: Harvard.

"Rabbi Among the Mechanics"

Gustafson, J.P. (1995). *The Dilemmas of Brief Therapy*. New York: Plenum.
Shapiro, E. (2001) *Eye Movement Desensitization and Reprocessing*, 2nd Ed. New York: Guilford.
van der Kolk et.al. (1996). *Traumatic Stress*. New York: Guilford.

"What Does Suffering Do?"

Duff, K. (1993). *The Alchemy of Illness*. New York: Pantheon.
Kavanaugh, K., ed. (1987) *John of the Cross: Selected Writings*. Mahwah, NJ: Paulist Press.

"Psychotherapy After Mohammed Atta"

Barzun, J. (2000). *From Dawn to Decadence*. New York: HarperCollins.
Cushman, P. (1995). *Constructing the Self, Constructing America.* Reading, MA: Addison-Wesley.
Horney, K. (1937). *The Neurotic Personality of Our Time*. New York: W. W. Norton.
Jung, C. G. (1953). *Two Essays on Analytical Psychology (Collected Works, Vol. 7)*. Princeton: Bollingen.

"The Domestication of the Truth"

Agee, J. (2000). *Let Us Now Praise Famous Men*. New York: Houghton Mifflin.

"The Owl Stick"

Norman, H., trans. (1982). *The Wishing Bone Cycle: Narrative Poems of the Swampy Cree Indians*. Santa Barbara, CA: Ross-Erikson.

ACKNOWLEDGMENTS

Self-absorbed as he often was, William Butler Yeats still had the sense to write, "My glory was that I had such friends." Amen. These friends I wish to glorify in detail, hence I am placing these thank-you's here in the back.

Most acknowledgments end with the typists. I will begin with them, since their hands and brains processed these essays more completely than anyone but myself. I hand-write first drafts. Hope Martin put the first half of my work onto disk. If she hadn't noticed a copy of Krishnamurti lying on my desk and started a conversation about it, I might never have dared to begin. One doesn't trust one's heart with just anyone. Another extraordinary person, Roma Naras, picked up where Hope left off. She has been accurate and prompt despite having many more important things to think about.

Voices had three editors during the period chronicled in this book. Edward Tick first published me. William Kir-Stimon took an active and ongoing interest in my work, and Monique Savlin has continued it.

Psychiatric Times' founder and editor-in-chief, John Schwartz, was willing to publish my unknown, dissenting voice (my AAP friend, Robbie Green, showed him a manuscript) at what I hope was the absolute nadir of psychotherapy's influence within psychiatry—despite the fact that therapists don't buy advertising space. During my tenure, Arline Kaplan and then Christine Potvin have been cheerful, level-headed managing editors at the *Times*.

Two university professors have read my work closely over the years and offered encouragement and discouragement, honestly and usefully. One is a dear friend, sociologist Brian Powers of the University of California, San Francisco. The other I met face-to-face only once, 18 years ago: psychiatrist and theorist James Paul Gustafson of the University of Wisconsin.

I have been sustained by a professional family consisting of several leaderless peer supervision/therapy groups (both here in Maine and in

195

the American Academy of Psychotherapists), as well as other fellow therapists with whom I have shared walks, breakfasts, and such like. The spirits and insights of all these kinfolk have found their way into these essays: Janice Arbarbanel, Ron Bailyn, Chris Beach, Peg Beehan, Walter Christie, Craig Cleaves, Enes Conadera, Grace Dickstein, Steve Feierstein, Sandy Hutton, Joan Larkin, Rick Lynch, Thomas Marino (who took the cover photograph), Margaret Nichols, John Rhead (who wrote the foreword for the Dorrance edition) Howard Rosenfield, Steve Sabom, Bruce St. Thomas, Janet Telford-Tyler, Beth Van Gorden, Karen Westerman, the late Joe Wolf, Jane Wood, and John Wortley.

I owe special gratitude to a pair of senior mentors who stuck with me through many periods of discouragement: Darrell Dawson and Leston Havens.

My psychiatric resident supervisees from Maine Medical Center, and a few other therapists who have sought supervision with me, are not named here. They know who they are and how stimulating and inspiring they have been for me.

Serious writers wish for editors and publishers who understand and are interested in what we are trying to say, and then help us to say it better. Instead we usually find salesmen, who wish to extract buzzwords that can then be spun to the various known markets. At Dorrance, Mary Beth Papciak served all conceivable functions in assisting me to produce a serviceable book whose success was in part a result of strong support from the American Academy of Psychotherapists. That success helped to attract the attention of The Analytic Press, where Paul Stepansky and Eleanor Starke Kobrin continued Mary Beth's work from their much stronger position. Dr. Stepansky's close reading and even closer philosophical questioning made me conscious of implicit themes that emerge most clearly from the book as a whole, rather than from the parts as they were (often hurriedly) written. He helped me to see what *The Thaw* was really about and chose a new subtitle to emphasize that.

And now to the most important of all. My family. Noel, Rosalie, Peter, and Marie make life worth living. Noel, my wife, has typically been the first to read any new piece, and her nontherapist's perspective has been invaluable in writing and in life. My parents, Grace and Fiori Genova, gave to me their enduring fascination with people and any sense of humor I may possess.

196

T - #0553 - 101024 - C0 - 229/152/11 - PB - 9780881633801 - Gloss Lamination